Wisdom Leadership

Health Science ~~Centers~~

LEADING POSITIVE CHANGE

Edited by

MARGARET PLEWS-OGAN

MD, MS
University of Virginia School of Medicine
Charlottesville, VA, USA

and

GENE BEYT

MD, MS
Heller School for Social Policy & Management
Brandeis University
Waltham, MA, USA

CULTURE, CONTEXT AND QUALITY IN HEALTH SCIENCES
RESEARCH, EDUCATION, LEADERSHIP AND PATIENT CARE
Series Editors
THOMAS S. INUI AND RICHARD M. FRANKEL

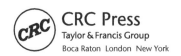

CRC Press
Taylor & Francis Group
Boca Raton London New York

CRC Press is an imprint of the
Taylor & Francis Group, an **informa** business

Contents

Contents

Acknowledgment

The editors would like to acknowledge Donna Kulawiak, Donna Burgett, and Jane Beyt for their wonderful support and editorial assistance.

Preface: Finding the Thread

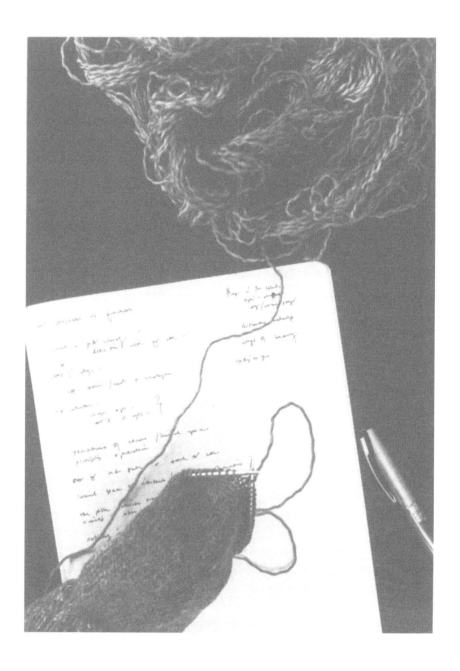

The Way It Is

There's a thread you follow. It goes among

things that change. But it doesn't change.

People wonder about what you are pursuing.

You have to explain about the thread.

But it is hard for others to see.

While you hold it you can't get lost.

Tragedies happen; people get hurt

or die; and you suffer and get old.

Nothing you do can stop time's unfolding.

You don't ever let go of the thread.

—William Stafford

In Greek mythology, Ariadne gave Theseus a ball of thread to help him find his way out of the Minotaur's labyrinth.

When we, the editors of the five volumes in this series on enhancing the professional culture of academic health science centers, gathered in Oxford, England, to talk about the series, we first had to ask ourselves, "Why do we feel a need to do this series, at this time?" We had come together with a sense of urgency, a sense that something was amiss in the world of health care, and we felt a need to respond. We also had a collective feeling of something deeper at work in this endeavor, and sensed that discovering these deeper forces at work among us would be key to writing these books well. Being students of meaning, aim, and purpose, we asked ourselves *the Five Whys*. Here is what we discovered about what was motivating us to be in that room and to recognize the need to change the culture of our academic health science centers. We want to deserve the trust our patients and our students have in us.

"Why?"

Because we have a moral compact

"Why?"

We are empowered to make certain changes

"Why?"

There are inherent privileges in doctoring and in health care and therefore our profession has a duty
"Why?"
This is necessary for a civil and just society
"Why?"
The advance of humankind

The changes that all of the series authors felt were so necessary in health care were grounded in the deepest part of ourselves as human beings, and in our desire to be truly our best selves as health-care professionals, and to have our health systems honor, reflect, and enhance our human connection and our collective human aspirations.

These are indeed challenging times. The business of health care has co-opted our intentions as healers and we have, to a greater or lesser degree, lost our way in the conflicting goals of our current work. The thread that grounds us as human beings, and that represents the very best of who we are and who we strive to be, is the same thread that grounds us in our healing profession. This thread is what connects us to one another in the best possible way. Patient-centered care is really about finding the thread that connects us as human beings with our patients. Compassion, meaning, gratitude, joy, these are all aspects of that thread that we share.

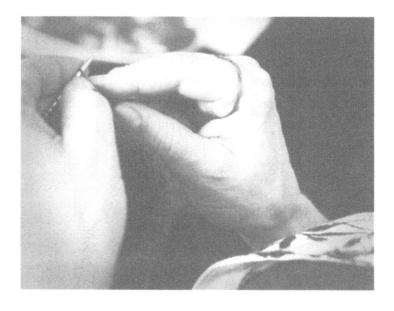

Wisdom is a concept that represents the ultimate in human capabilities. In Erikson's stages of human development, wisdom characterizes the final and pinnacle stage.[*] It represents the best of who we can be as human beings. If wisdom is the ultimate in human development then it also represents the ultimate in our development as a community charged with the most awesome of tasks, that of caring for and protecting the lives of others. This book on leadership is all about how we, as leaders, can foster capacities that can help us, and our health-care communities, to be our best selves, together.

Margaret Plews-Ogan
Gene Beyt
August 2013

---

[*]   Erikson, Erik. *Identity and the Life Cycle*. New York, NY: Norton and Company; 1980.

List of Contributors

Monika Ardelt, PhD
Associate Professor, Department of Sociology and Criminology, Faculty in the Center for Spirituality and Health, University of Florida

Gene Beyt, MD, MS
Visiting Scholar, Heller School for Social Policy and Management, Brandeis University

Dorrie K. Fontaine, RN, PhD
Professor and Dean, School of Nursing, University of Virginia

Richard M. Frankel, PhD
Professor of Medicine and Geriatrics, Senior Research Scientist, Regenstrief Institute, Indiana University School of Medicine

Al Gatmaitan, MHA
Chief Executive Officer, Indiana University Health Arnett

Jody Hoffer Gittell, PhD
Professor, Executive Director, Relational Coordination Research Collaborative, Heller School for Social Policy and Management, Brandeis University

Matthew Goodman, MD
Associate Professor of Medicine, Division of General Medicine, Geriatrics and Palliative Care, University of Virginia School of Medicine

Julie Haizlip, MD
Associate Professor of Pediatrics and Anesthesia, University of Virginia School of Medicine

Thomas S. Inui, ScM, MD
Director of Research, Indiana University Center for Global Health, Professor of Medicine, Indiana University School of Medicine, Investigator, Regenstrief Institute

Ann Kellams, MD
Associate Professor of Pediatrics, Healer's Art Program, University of Virginia School of Medicine

Bryce Kellams, MD
Assistant Clinical Professor of Family Medicine, Healer's Art Program, University of Virginia School of Medicine

Sylvester N. Kimaiyo
Chief Executive Officer, Indiana University–Kenya AMPATH (Academic Model for Providing Access to Healthcare)

Curt Lindberg, DMan, MHA
Director, Partnership for Complex Systems and Healthcare Innovation, Billings Clinic, Principal, Partners in Complexity

Robert Lindberg, MD
Clinical Instructor of Medicine, Columbia University College of Physicians and Surgeons

Beth A. Lown, MD
Associate Professor of Medicine, Harvard Medical School, Medical Director, The Schwartz Center for Compassionate Healthcare

Joe Mamlin, MD
AMPATH (Academic Model for Providing Access to Healthcare) Field Director, Faculty of Health Sciences, Moi University, Kenya, and Professor Emeritus of Medicine, Indiana University School of Medicine

Angela Barron McBride, PhD, RN
Distinguished Professor and University Dean Emerita, Indiana University School of Nursing

Sara Nadelman, MPH
Former manager, Center for Professionalism and Peer Support, Brigham and Women's Hospital, Harvard Medical School

Jim Ogan, MD
Associate Professor of Pediatrics, University of Virginia

Ora Hirsch Pescovitz, MD
Executive Vice President for Medical Affairs, Chief Executive Officer, Health System, Professor, Pediatric Endocrinology, University of Michigan

Margaret Plews-Ogan, MD, MS
Associate Professor of Medicine, Chief, Division of General Medicine, Geriatrics and Palliative Medicine, Director, University of Virginia School of Medicine's Center for Appreciative Practice

List of Contributors

Cynda H. Rushton, RN, PhD
Professor of Clinical Ethics, School of Nursing, Johns Hopkins University, Program Director, Harriet Lane Compassionate Care Program, The Johns Hopkins Children's Center, Johns Hopkins Berman Institute of Ethics

Michele Saysana, MD
Assistant Professor of Clinical Pediatrics, Indiana University School of Medicine, Medical Director of Quality and Safety, Riley Hospital for Children at Indiana University Health

John Schorling, MD, MPH
Professor of Medicine, Director Physician Wellness Program and Mindfulness Center, University of Virginia School of Medicine

John G. Scott, MD, PhD
Family Physician, Northeastern Vermont Regional Hospital, Assistant Professor of Family Medicine, Department of Family Medicine, Robert Wood Johnson Medical School

Jo Shapiro, MD
Associate Professor of Otology and Laryngology, Harvard Medical School and Chief of the Division of Otolaryngology, Director of the Center for Professionalism and Peer Support at Brigham and Women's Hospital

Monica Sharma, MD
Former Director, Leadership and Capacity Development, United Nations, Leadership Development for Sustainable Equitable Change, Tata Chair Professor, Tata Institute of Social Sciences, Mumbai

Wiley "Chip" Souba, MD, ScD, MBA
Vice-President for Health Affairs, Dean and Professor of Surgery, Geisel School of Medicine, Dartmouth College

Anthony L. Suchman, MD, MA
Clinical Professor of Medicine and Psychiatry, University of Rochester

Part 1

Wisdom and Leadership

Introduction

Leadership and Management in Two Different Cultures: "It's Not What You Say . . ."

Thomas S. Inui and Richard M. Frankel with S. N. Kimaiyo

I think, therefore I am (Cogito ergo sum).

—René Descartes

We are, therefore I am.

—African tribal saying

ON A SUNNY MONDAY MORNING EARLY IN JANUARY 2011, DR. SYLVESTER Kimaiyo, the presiding officer, chief executive officer (CEO), and program manager for the Indiana University–Kenya USAID-AMPATH (United States Agency for International Development–Academic Model for Providing Access to Healthcare) program, opened AMPATH's monthly "program operations meeting" by greeting everyone and wishing all those present in the rather large meeting room "Happy New Year!" This invoked an echoing response from everyone. Dr. Kimaiyo then ran through a 5-minute opening statement that touched lightly and good-heartedly on a number of major issues, including:

- the core mission of AMPATH, to serve vulnerable patients attempting to "live positively" with HIV
- the upcoming re-competition for the USAID core grant (the lifeblood of AMPATH's clinical program)
- the need to work harder than ever in the coming year—with the same resources as last year
- the observation that an AMPATH vehicle was rolled over last week, far away from any authorized route committed to operations
- the need to make every shilling count and to avoid "leakage"—with allusions to missing (and perhaps pilfered) medications.

Dr. Kimaiyo's opening statement was a *tour de force*. In the next hour all those present heard brief reports from more than 40 different AMPATH program unit managers, each of whom echoed Dr. Kimaiyo's New Year greeting (with a response of "Happy New Year!" each time from all those assembled—I (TSI) was thinking, "Can I get an amen?!"). Each presentation in its own way also reinforced a commitment to serve, to work harder, and to rise to challenges as the staff entered the new year.

After witnessing another of these program operations meetings in June 2011, a visiting CEO from a major academic medical center in North America whispered to Inui, "What in the world can these meetings accomplish?!" Any reasonable organizational consultant would observe quickly that there were far too many "direct reports" to Dr. Kimaiyo. He could hardly "manage" them all. It was also likely that no substantive briefing information about how to successfully manage the various programs could be conveyed to everyone in a 90-minute meeting. With no standard format for sharing information, what possible function could be served by having so many people travel to the monthly operations meeting from their individual localities and offices on a busy Monday morning?

After this June meeting, Dr. Kimayo provided a history of the weekly program operations meeting as part of his backgrounding for the North American CEO. He explained that in the beginning, late 2001, the meeting only involved the four AMPATH clinicians and it was used for them to meet once a week to discuss the few patients they were seeing. In those days "AMPATH" meant "Academic Model for Prevention and Treatment of HIV/AIDS" and the program provided care to only a few individuals in a hospital room borrowed from the Tuberculosis Clinic at the Moi Teaching and Referral Hospital. Standard therapeutic approaches for managing people with HIV/AIDS were being formulated. The four clinicians who participated in the weekly operations meeting—two physicians, a nurse, and a clinical officer (a physician's assistant)—needed to exchange information about particular patients, the response of these patients to antiretroviral drugs, and whether there were enough resources to start any additional patients on therapy.

As time passed, AMPATH grew rapidly, especially after international resources become available for financing complex regimens of antiretroviral drug therapy, expanding from the first patient in 2001 to more than 130 000 patients with HIV enrolled for care in the present-day program. With the increase in the number of individuals cared for by AMPATH also came greater numbers of staff, integration with Ministry of Health programs, and a broader array of health-supporting services, organized into AMPATH program units, each with its own leadership. These services included support of nutritional security, economic security (e.g., micro-enterprise "round robin loans"), legal services, services to orphans and widows, tuberculosis screening and treatment, community screening, and staff education for HIV/AIDS care. AMPATH's core program administrative and other services also increased in size and complexity, including those for electronic health record development, grants and contracts administration, data management, monitoring and evaluation, demonstration farms, human resources, and transportation pool services. AMPATH's program operations meeting also grew in size, from four participants to 10, then 20, then 30, and now more than 40. Because of the large number of personnel involved, the meeting was changed from weekly to monthly.

Along the way, AMPATH program manager Dr. Kimaiyo, and his close colleague Dr. Joseph Mamlin, the Indiana field program director, concluded that the program operations meeting had become too large to make meaningful contributions to top-level management. Divisions would have to emerge for the larger enterprise, and a "middle management" would have to be created. The program manager's monthly program operations meeting should give way to divisional meetings. An announcement was drafted and issued to all, canceling the program manager's program operations meetings. Each division could decide upon its own schedule of meetings, perhaps arranging to rotate the location across the geographic region in which the 53 AMPATH clinics and satellites now operated in western Kenya. A good decision had been made that would increase the efficiency of program management, or so Dr. Mamlin and Dr. Kimaiyo thought.

On the first Monday morning of the next month, Dr. Kimaiyo was in his office when a staff member came in to say, "Pardon, sir, but you should know that everyone is waiting for you in the operations meeting room!" Astonished, Dr. Kimaiyo walked down the hall to the large meeting room to discover that all of the 40-plus direct reports had traveled from everywhere in the AMPATH service area to assemble themselves—contrary to his explicit instructions—for the program operations meeting, whether or not it had been officially discontinued. "They just want to get together, see one another, hear one another's voices, and know that they are all in this together," Kimayo said. "It isn't only the information they present that's important. It is, in addition, that they feel and know one another's commitment to the enormous challenge we all face."

There is much to be learned from this story. We understand the functions of leadership and management to be many. What a leader says and does inspires, informs, incentivizes, aligns, articulates, and even occasionally commands. He or she is a "lightning rod" for issues and a barometer for changes in an organization's environment. A leader also convenes and encourages individuals to express their feelings, their passions, and their commitment to a cause. In a distributed leadership environment the few at the very top carry only a part of the "load." The larger community of leadership and line workers need to pull together (the Kiswahili word is *harambee*), hear one another's views, celebrate, mourn their losses, and envision, track, and map their progress together. Management is not simply a matter of receiving and processing the usual "facts" about program performance. Instead, it also includes sharing the highs and lows, the struggle, and even re-kindling a sense of common identity ("who we are").

Our notion of what a "chief executive officer" does in North America emphasizes the need for critical information (the "dashboard") and command decisions. *Cogito ergo sum*, a North American CEO might assert. While the AMPATH CEO surely does need to make certain decisions and commitments on behalf of all in his large program, he might say of the leadership tasks he faces in this crucial enterprise: "*We* are, therefore *I* am."

1

Wisdom is a Worthy Construct

Margaret Plews-Ogan and Monika Ardelt

SOMETIMES WE LEARN THINGS THE HARD WAY. IN THESE DIFFICULT experiences lie the seeds of wisdom, and the passion for change. Today, throughout our academic health science centers (AHSCs), there are passionate change agents, leaders at all levels who are championing change, propelled by wisdom gained from deep and sometimes painful experience. Let me introduce you to Dr. Smith. He is a well-respected pediatric surgeon at a large academic health center who was caring for a very sick child in the intensive care unit. The child was deteriorating. The nurse working on the team had concerns that the child was developing sepsis despite receiving multiple antibiotics. Dr. Smith discounted the nurse's concerns. It turned out the nurse was right, and a few days later the child died of overwhelming fungal sepsis. Dr. Smith was devastated, feeling that perhaps had he picked up the condition earlier the child might have lived. In a conversation now 10 years later, Dr. Smith relates this experience as being truly transformative in his development. He points to learning to recognize his limitations, to acknowledge uncertainty and imperfection, to communicate well as a team, and to really be able and willing to both speak up and listen to truly help one another, all things he didn't learn in medical school. As he put it: "I never knew how we could, with a real team, help fix each other's failings, one step at a time." Today, Dr. Smith teaches his students and residents about humility, listening, and the critical nature of teamwork. In the process, he is leading a change in health care.

Change is in the wind, or, as Kenneth Cohn *et al.*[1] reflected, the tectonic plates are shifting in AHSCs. Over the past 10 years, there has been a clarion call for attention to the organizational culture of the AHSC, the environment in which our patients are cared for and our students, residents, and fellows are trained.[2–6] There is now broad recognition that the organizational culture exerts profound influences on patient care, successful research, and appropriate training, and our organizational culture is not what we all want it to be.[7–15] Dr. Smith learned the hard way about the limits of knowledge and the importance of true teamwork. He had to find his own way to talk about mistakes openly and learn from them. He had to figure out on his own how first to abandon his "lone captain of the ship" mentality and reconfigure his self-understanding as a member of a highly functioning team. As they learned from this difficult experience, Dr. Smith and his team members were creating a new culture in their AHSC.

Although this book is about leadership, it is really about wisdom. It is about fostering wise leaders and leaders fostering wisdom in our health-care organizations and in our health professional schools. Why wisdom? In the paragraphs that follow we briefly recall some of the more important calls for change in our health-care systems. These calls for change have strikingly similar themes: they call for a culture of compassion, other-centeredness and self-awareness, relationality and collaboration, teamwork, embracing complexity, applying knowledge to discern the right action, and a refocusing on the greater good. Consider for a moment the characteristics generally associated with wise persons. Our definition of wisdom reflects most of the commonly accepted attributes of wise persons, including *understanding the deeper meaning of things, knowing the limits of knowledge, tolerating ambiguity, engaging in reflective and self-reflective thinking, showing compassion and sympathy toward others, and the capacity to be other-centered.*[16,17] Perhaps wisdom is a helpful construct to frame our discussion about the culture of health care. As William Branch and Gary Mitchell[18] suggest, "wisdom is what we should be striving for in our development as clinicians . . . seeking wisdom should be embedded in our culture."

The basic premises of this book on leadership and the culture of AHSCs are:
- wisdom is a worthy and helpful construct to have in mind when considering both what kind of culture we want to foster in the AHSC and what leadership capacities are critical to fostering this culture
- wisdom can be attained through fostering the capacities inherent in all of us
- wisdom is both intra- and interpersonal; it happens in community, in a matrix that leaders at all levels help to create.

Each of the chapters in this book reflects a key component of wisdom and a critical capacity in nurturing wisdom in individuals and organizations. Each chapter also tells a story of leadership.

Calls for Change

Let us begin first with a look at where we are at this moment of tremendous change, the "tectonic plate shift" to which Cohn *et al.*[1] refer and the forces behind that shift.

The Institute of Medicine report *Academic Health Centers: Leading Change in the 21st Century* (2004) notes that health care is changing in fundamental ways.[4] Propelled by the stark reality of preventable errors in medical care, a new focus on quality and patient safety brings front and center the need for standardization, teamwork, and safer systems that take into account our human fallibility. Major advances in the care of previously fatal diseases now demand a shift in attention from acute care to chronic illness management, and the race is turning from hare to tortoise. Financial constraints and competition have resulted in an ever-higher bar for efficiency and cost-effectiveness, and at times it seems that the business of health care has torn us from our roots of altruism and the greater good. The human genome project has added marvelous complexity to our one-size-fits-all approach to both prevention and treatment of disease. With shrinking research dollars and increasing complexity, success in research now demands high degrees of collaboration (team science) to achieve translational goals and to leverage the interdisciplinary perspectives needed to approach complex scientific questions. The education of health-care professionals, we now recognize, must be a collaborative, interprofessional process in an environment that models the best of quality, efficiency, and patient-centeredness. Finally, in challenging economic times with an ever-increasing population of uninsured and underinsured, the role of the AHSC in improving the health of the population, not just the population with health insurance, may require a whole new paradigm.

These all represent major, fundamental shifts in the tasks of the AHSC. To meet these demands the report calls on the AHSC to develop leaders at all levels who can, among other things, improve integration and foster cooperation across the AHSC enterprise and improve health by providing guidance on pressing societal problems.[4]

In 2003, the Commonwealth Fund Taskforce on Academic Health Centers (AHCs) released a report that delineated the challenges and opportunities facing AHCs in this time of change and what the future might look like as they transform to meet these challenges.

> To cope with increasing change and uncertainty, AHC collectively and individually, must be able to learn quickly and act expeditiously. This will require changes in institutional culture that increase openness, teamwork, commitment to learning, continuous improvement, accountability and patient-centeredness. Transforming the culture of AHCs is likely to be a lengthy and complex process.[19]

Culture and Safety

Beginning with the Institute of Medicine's report *To Err is Human*,[20] health care has been challenged with the stark reality of human error. We have made progress,[21] but we have yet to achieve a culture in which human fallibility is recognized and mitigated, errors are openly acknowledged, and continuous learning is a priority. Physicians are still trained in an environment where mistakes are not discussed, where perfection is the implicit expectation, where disclosure of error is neither taught nor consistently practiced, and where peer support for dealing with errors is not available. A culture of safety in health care is one that supports inquiry rather than judgment, openness rather than secrecy, a flat hierarchy with engagement of all members of the team, and a continuous awareness of what one does not know and what could go wrong. By all measures we are far from that goal.[22–25]

Culture and Meaning

In 2007 Darryl Kirch[2] used his Association of American Medical Colleges presidential address to remind us that "we have the possibility of creating a much more meaningful and gratifying culture for our faculty, staff and learners, and especially for the patients we have committed to serve." He commented on how distressed we have all felt by the gap between what we actually have been doing in practice and the care we know we should deliver. Resolution of that distress, he suggested, will come when we can finally align how we are with how we want to be and the environment and culture in which we find ourselves with our deeply held values.

Culture and Professionalism

Thomas Inui,[3] in *A Flag in the Wind,* his Association of American Medical Colleges monograph on education for professionalism, notes that the medical profession is challenged by an erosion of the public's trust. Entangled in health care as big business, health-care professionals' motivations have become suspect. Patients and families perceive that our focus in health care has been on techno-logical advances, perhaps at the expense of compassion.

> My own belief is that the present intensity of our discourse about profession-alism in medicine represents both a flight from commercialism, on the one hand, and a corresponding need to reaffirm our deeper values and reclaim our authenticity as trusted healers, on the other.[3]

> There can be no simple or simple-minded response to the question of how to begin to change the environment in which our students learn and what profes-sionals hold dear and seek to exemplify in their actions. If the most powerful learning is experiential, and students are close observers of the scene in aca-demic health centers, essentially we as faculty are challenged to change what we think, say, and do as individuals and as members of a community.[3]

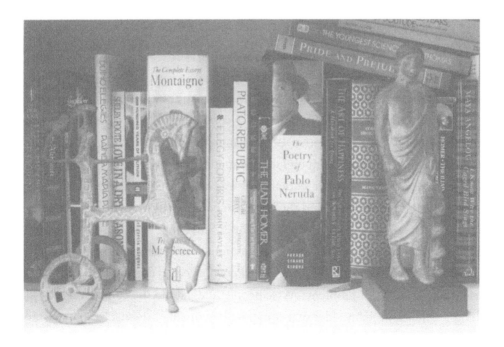

Wisdom: A Concept Worth Thinking About

Wisdom is not a concept that is frequently discussed in the context of health care. What is wisdom, and how might wisdom be a framework for our thinking about the capacities we wish to foster in the AHSCs?

Philosophers' Long Engagement with Wisdom

At the beginning of the philosophical tradition of Western culture, Socrates and Plato formulated ideas that still guide us today when we think about wisdom.[26] One of the most important is the distinction between wisdom as an understanding of the ultimate nature of things (Sophia) and practical wisdom (Phronesis)—that is, knowing the best course of action and resisting the undue influence of the emotions. Socrates also gave us the notion of humility as essential to wisdom: the person who is continually aware of what he or she does not know is wiser than one who does not know the limits of their knowledge.[27] A bit later, Aristotle emphasized that to be wise was to strive for moral excellence and wisdom is therefore tied to moral behavior.[28,29] It would be centuries later that the concept of wisdom was brought forward as a subject worthy of scientific exploration. Wisdom is a difficult topic for science, and it is only recently that psychology and sociology have taken on the challenge.

Implicit Theories of Wisdom

In the past 30 years, psychologists and sociologists have accumulated insights from their research about wisdom. Vivian Clayton and Julie Birren[30] in the 1980s did some of the earliest scientific investigations of wisdom. Their research into people's common understanding of wisdom showed that it is considered multidimensional and integrative, combining emotion as well as intellect. The affective dimension of wisdom included empathy, understanding, peacefulness, and gentleness. The reflective component was characterized by the qualities of introspection and intuition, and the cognitive component by knowledge, experience, intellect, pragmatism, and observation.[30] Since that time, wisdom research has continued to demonstrate its multidimensional nature. Other research[31] characterizes wise persons as having deep knowledge and the ability to apply that knowledge to difficult problems. Wise people understand the complex nature of things, can look at many sides of a situation, be critical of themselves, and avoid quick judgments. They are concerned about others and can transcend their own self-interest to consider the concerns of others.

Wisdom versus Intelligence

Is wisdom the same as intelligence? Robert Sternberg's[32] work suggests it is not. According to him, intelligence seeks knowledge and uses what is known. Wisdom, on the other hand, seeks to *grasp the deeper meaning* of what is known and to *understand the limits of knowledge*. Wisdom resists automatic thinking *and seeks to understand ambiguity better*, whereas *intelligence seeks to eliminate ambiguity*. Other researchers confirm distinct differences between perceptions of wisdom and intelligence, with wisdom encompassing self-reflection and self-knowledge, altruism and empathy.[33]

Wisdom has also been associated with how people make big life decisions. Qualities of wisdom include knowledge about human nature, strategies for dealing with life conflicts, being able to balance individual and common good, and recognizing and managing uncertainty.[34,35]

Wisdom and the Common Good

How do wise persons actually go about making these difficult decisions? How do they balance competing values? What guides them in making these complex decisions? What guides the decisions of a wise leader like Nelson Mandela versus a leader like Hitler who, although arguably an intelligent leader, would never be considered wise? One answer is that it is the notion of *the common good* that distinguishes wise decisions. In this application of intelligence and experience, wise people have to balance intra-, inter-, and extrapersonal interests and be able to juggle both short- and long-term views, all guided by the ultimate value of achieving the common good.[36,37]

Ardelt's Three-Dimensional Wisdom Model

Monika Ardelt[17] integrated the cognitive, reflective and compassionate aspects of wisdom into a three-dimensional (3-D) wisdom model. Returning to the concept first brought forth by Clayton and Birren[30] that wisdom is an integration of cognitive, reflective, and affective components, Ardelt[38] states "wisdom does not simply refer to a 'state of knowledge' but to a *process* or *state of being*. Wisdom cannot necessarily be found in what a person says but is expressed through an individual's personality and conduct in life." Ardelt's 3-D model of wisdom is presented here as one that captures the multidimensional nature of wisdom and can serve as a basis for wisdom development in AHSCs.

TABLE 1.1 A Three-Dimensional Wisdom Model

Dimension	Definition
Cognitive	An understanding of life and a desire to know the truth—that is, to comprehend the significance and deeper meaning of phenomena and events, particularly with regard to intra- and interpersonal matters
	Includes knowledge and acceptance of the positive and negative aspects of human nature, of the inherent limits of knowledge, and of life's unpredictability, uncertainties, and complexities
Reflective	A perception of phenomena and events from multiple perspectives
	Requires self-examination, self-awareness, and self-insight
Compassionate	All-encompassing sympathetic and compassionate love accompanied by a motivation to foster the well-being of all
	Requires the transcendence of self-centeredness

Note: adapted from Ardelt[17]

As outlined in Table 1.1, Ardelt describes the *cognitive dimension of wisdom* as a desire to know the deeper truth and meaning about life, particularly as it relates to the intrapersonal and interpersonal facets of life. This includes knowledge and acceptance of the positive and negative aspects of human nature, of the inherent limits of knowledge and of life's unpredictability and uncertainties. The *reflective component of wisdom* represents self-examination, self-awareness, self-insight, and the ability to look at phenomena and events from different perspectives. This reflective component is seen as essential to the development of wisdom, because it allows people to reflect on their experience—to learn, change, and grow wiser. Reflection also protects us from becoming entrenched in a particular stance, as it promotes our consideration of things from multiple perspectives, reducing our self-centeredness, and helping us to become aware of and ultimately transcend our own fears, biases, and projections. The *compassionate dimension of wisdom* manifests as sympathetic and compassionate love for others, which increases as self-centeredness is transcended.

In summary, a wise person is one who is compassionate and other-centered, understands complexity and the deeper meaning of things, avoids black-and-white thinking, can tolerate ambiguity, is aware of the limitations of knowledge, is self-reflective and capable of seeing things from many different perspectives, learns from experiences and the experiences and perspectives of others, and is guided by the common, ultimate good.

Wisdom as Our Inherent Being: "Our Best Selves"

Warren Kinghorn[39] wrote an important article on professionalism and medical education in which he makes the distinction between *techne*, or technical knowledge, and *phronesis*, or practical wisdom. Professionalism in health care is not only about *techne*, as health care is not a product separate from who we are as doctors or nurses. It is more about character than about knowledge, for it has to do with how we apply knowledge to right action, in whatever circumstance we find ourselves. Aristotle's notion of *eudemonia* or human flourishing has imbedded in it the understanding that all humans have a natural orientation toward the good, but we do not necessarily know how to achieve the good. Rather, we need to experience it through a process of education, which includes mentoring and practice or habit. This practice differentiates moral excellence and eventually leads to *arete*, or virtue. According to Kinghorn[39]:

> Unless physicians are the sorts of persons who, through a lifetime of practice and habituation, have cultivated excellence of practical wisdom by formation in particular types of moral communities, the precepts will probably be useless; and furthermore, if practical wisdom is present, the precepts will probably be unnecessary. The practically wise person doesn't need general guidelines about how to act morally; the practically unwise person cannot successfully apply such guidelines when they are given.

Thus if we are to foster wisdom in health professionals, it is a matter that reaches far beyond imparting knowledge. Our attention in the AHSCs must be focused on deeper forces that shape the matrix in which health professionals learn and which are manifest in the way we are with one another and with our patients. These deeper forces are particularly visible when challenges arise and we respond to those challenges with our deeper selves.

Critical Incidents and Wisdom Development

Ardelt[40] has studied how wisdom is manifest in the ways people respond to challenging circumstances. Are there critical situations in which wisdom is more likely to develop, situations particularly primed for the development of wisdom? (In education we might call these "teachable moments," in leadership, "trigger events.") If so, the way the individual is supported or how the organization responds in these critical situations may have lasting repercussions, either positive or negative.

Wisdom from Adversity: Medical Error as Critical Incident

Adversity can be a powerful teacher of wisdom. Judith Glück et al.[41] used narrative to study the development of wisdom. They asked subjects to describe a situation in which they acted wisely, a situation in which they acted foolishly, and a "peak experience" situation. Analyzing the narratives, they found that *wisdom stories* more often involved *difficult* life situations or negative events, implying that wisdom perhaps develops through the experience of adversity. Juan Pascual-Leone et al.[42] described these challenging situations as "ultimate limit situations," circumstances that "cannot be undone and are nonetheless faced with consciousness and resolve . . . situations like death, illness, aging, . . . absolute failure . . . uncontrollable fear." He suggests that confronting these situations with awareness and resolve can lead to remarkable growth in the self and the natural emergence of the transcendent self, "if they do not destroy the person first."[42] Researchers studying posttraumatic growth suggest that trauma induces a disruption in our understanding of ourselves and the world (our schema) and that disruption forces us to rework our understanding of ourselves and the world, resulting in learning and growth with the potential for wisdom as the final result.[43,44]

Arthur Kleinman[45] gives clear voice to the heart of this matter. Inarguably one of the leading writers and thinkers of our time, Kleinman, in the wake of his wife's death, found himself "quite literally lost." Searching for insight and wisdom, he found himself going back to the philosophical challenges that had captivated him at the beginning of his career. But this time he understood his quest for wisdom differently. "I needed an intellectual interlocutor who could come right down into my experience and illuminate it from within." At that moment, it was William James[46] whose words struck home.

> If this life be not a real fight, in which something is eternally gained for the universe by success, it is no better than a game of private theatricals from which one may withdraw at will. But it feels like a real fight, as if there were something really wild in the universe which we, with all our idealities and faithfulnesses, are needed to redeem.

Kleinman[45] writes about this critical juncture in his life.

> The wisdom I needed came out of my readiness to respond to James's push-
> ing at a certain time when I was faced with a problem central to the human
> condition: a problem that connected me up with the grain of life and with the
> existential uncertainty of our being. Wisdom needs to be experienced to be
> effective, and is effective not as an idea, but as a lived feeling and a moral prac-
> tice that redeems our humanness amid inevitable disappointment and defeat.

Research by Plews-Ogan *et al.*[47] on the Wisdom in Medicine project suggests
that a serious medical error can be a situation that catalyzes positive change
and the development of wisdom in physicians. These profoundly challenging
experiences change doctors, for better or for worse. There are ways to potentially
foster wisdom in these circumstances. Participants related that being able to talk
about the experience, support from colleagues, disclosure, forgiveness, and making positive changes were all helpful in their moving through this experience in
a positive way.[48,49] If we are to foster wisdom in our AHSCs, we must attend to
how we respond, individually and collectively, when things go wrong. Creating an
environment of openness, honesty, curiosity, a desire to learn (rather than judgment and blame), and support gives the community the best chance for wisdom
and growth. Consider how Dr. Smith, whom we introduced at the beginning of
this chapter, would have benefitted had he had a safe, supportive environment
in which to discuss his mistake!

Wisdom and Situations of Moral Conflict

Wisdom is not static and is best recognized in the context of complex ambiguous situations, many of which involve conflicting values. As wisdom researchers,
Ursula Staudinger and Judith Glück[50] point out that wisdom concerns the "mastery of dialectics: dialectics between good and bad . . . certainty and doubt . . .
selfishness and altruism," and wisdom "embraces the contradictions in life and
draws insight from them." Wisdom researcher John Meacham[51] suggests that this
balancing between knowing and doubting is perhaps a defining characteristic of
wisdom: "The essence of wisdom is to hold the attitude that knowledge is fallible
and to strive for a balance between knowing and doubting." Kinghorn[39] believes
that professionalism (or what he suggests is practical wisdom) is best taught in a
setting where the truth of two conflicting values is exposed and where students

are able to see and practice wise action in these complex settings. "Moral excellence is often found in the in-between of two vices." For example, between recklessness and cowardice one finds courage.[39] Leaders who seek to develop capacities for wisdom in the community must attend particularly to those critical incident situations that present complexity and moral conflict, and foster an atmosphere in which that ambiguity can be openly acknowledged and explored, and too-confident knowing avoided.

The Change Starts with Each of Us: Fostering Capacities of Wisdom and Leading from Where We Are

Wiley Souba[52] has proposed a new ontological model of leadership as a *way of being* rather than something outside ourselves that we learn (as we shall see in Chapter 10). He focuses on language as a vehicle for "seeing things differently," and that ability to see things differently then opens the opportunity for right action and leading from what he calls our natural self-expression. In an *Academic Medicine* article from 2011, he leads us toward an awareness of how our mental model shapes our reality and how we can, through self-awareness, self-reflection, and language, reshape that mental model and, therefore, reshape our reality for the better.[53] He goes on to suggest that our language needs to change if we are to foster the development of our best selves.

> Only by means of the language of leadership can you and I *cultivate and nurture ourselves and others, each and every day, to become the wiser, more enlightened and more evolved human beings that we are intended to become.* Only through language can we create and use that discerning wisdom to solve the world's problems prudently and compassionately and in so doing contribute to global transformation. We are the languagers of our future. Let us not pass on that opportunity to be homo sapiens, *to be wise people.* It is both a responsibility and a privilege.[53]

Fostering Wisdom

All of this has implications for how one might foster wisdom in individuals or organizations. It suggests that our attention should be focused on fostering *capacities* in people that cultivate wisdom and *creating a context* in which these capacities can be honed, refined, and practiced. Leading then becomes more a process of fostering those capacities in all of us, individually and collectively, to "become the wiser, more enlightened and evolved beings we are intended to become"[53] and to create a context in which we, and our trainees, can *grow up wise*.

Ubuntu (We are, therefore I am): Fostering Wisdom in Community

Meacham[51] makes the point that wisdom really does begin not in our own individual heads but rather in interpersonal relationships. He points out that wisdom is learned and maintained in community, in an interpersonal matrix.

> The maintenance of wisdom throughout the life course and its restoration if it has been lost depends upon the continued immersion of the individual within a *wisdom atmosphere* that assists the individual in avoiding the extremes of too confident knowing and of paralyzing doubt. In a wisdom atmosphere, there is a supportive network of interpersonal relations in which doubts, uncertainties and questions can be openly expressed, in which ambiguities and contradictions can be tolerated, so that individuals are not forced to adopt the defensive position of too confident knowing. Furthermore, the recognition through expressing one's doubts that others share similar doubts and yet have found a basis for confident action can keep individuals from being forced into the position of paralyzing skepticism.[51]

If that is the case, what does fostering wisdom look like in a community?

Fostering a "Wisdom Atmosphere" in the Academic Health Science Center

Using Ardelt's 3-D model of wisdom as a conceptual framework (*see* Table 1.1), we can begin to identify *wisdom-related capacities* and how they might be fostered to create what Meacham describes as a wisdom atmosphere in our AHSCs. In the chapters that follow, authors describe ways in which they, as formal or informal leaders, have fostered these capacities within their AHSC communities. Their accounts reflect the wisdom components in Ardelt's 3-D model of wisdom.

The *cognitive component of wisdom* in Ardelt's model includes the *capacity to see the deeper meaning and significance of things*, including knowledge of the positive and negative aspects of human nature, the inherent limits of knowledge and of life's unpredictability, uncertainties, and complexity. In Chapter 2, Anne and Bryce Kellams describe their experience in fostering meaning in the AHSC. Fortunately for those of us in health care, our work has deep and intrinsic meaning. Unfortunately, too often we lose sight of that deeper meaning in our quest for fiscal solvency, efficiency, and our business orientation. Another feature of the cognitive component of wisdom is understanding and embracing complexity. Curt Lindberg and colleagues describe in Chapter 8 their experiences with complexity science and fostering a community's *capacity to deal with complexity*. Another cognitive feature of wisdom is the *capacity for humility*, or understanding and accepting the limits of knowledge. In Chapter 4, Jo Shapiro and Sara Nadelman describe a powerfully successful program of peer support that creates a wisdom atmosphere where medical mistakes can be openly acknowledged, the myth of the all-knowing perfect physician is dispelled, and learning, growth, and trust are fostered in the wake of an error.

The *reflective component of wisdom* refers to the individual or collective capacity to reflect on the self, see things from different perspectives, and rise above one's own fears and projections. Monika Ardelt considers this *capacity for self-reflection* to be essential for individuals or organizations to grow in wisdom. In Wiley Souba's[53] model, this capacity would enable a leader to be aware of their mindset and therefore to be free to reshape it. This can also happen in community, and leaders can intentionally foster this process in themselves and in the communities they lead. In Chapter 3, John Schorling and Matthew Goodman relate their experiences of bringing mindfulness to an AHSC as a means of enhancing its capacity for reflection. In Chapter 7, Julie Haizlip and Margaret Plews-Ogan describe the use of appreciative practices as a means of creating a collective intentional focus on the positive in our organizations and in ourselves.

The *compassionate component of wisdom* is made up of the capacity for sympathetic and compassionate love. One might think that health-care organizations would be deeply infused with compassionate love, given the nature of the work that they do. But as all of us know who work in health care, our organizations are sometimes anything but compassionate. In Chapter 5, Dorrie Fontaine and colleagues relate their experience of reinfusing the AHSC with compassion and *fostering compassion* in all facets of the organization.

Underlying all of this is the capacity for relationship, the community matrix in which these capacities are formed. In Chapter 6, Jody Hoffer Gittell and

Anthony Suchman describe their work in fostering relationship-centeredness in the AHSCs.

Wisdom as Seeking the Greater Good: The Academic Health Science Center and Society

Wisdom is fundamentally rooted in discerning and acting for the common good. Robert Sternberg[54] points out "Wisdom is in large part a decision to use one's intelligence, creativity and knowledge for a common good. Thus, wisdom involves not only skills in the use of these elements but also the disposition to use them for the common good." If what Tom Inui[3] asserts is true, the call for change in our AHSCs to enhance the professional culture has something to do with our desire to be part of a worthy and trusted group of healers, teachers, and researchers, whose work is not for personal gain but to improve the health of the patient and the community (be that local or global). If the AHSC wants to be that trusted group whose work is not suspect and whose opinion is considered pure in focus, then its goal must be to represent that common good in all that it does. We need wise leaders, but in an environment as complex as our AHSC we need *lots* of wisdom, in all parts of our organizations. And we need a matrix, a *wisdom atmosphere*, in which to train our students and treat our patients. This book is about creating that matrix, and it is filled with stories of leaders at all levels, formal and informal, who are creating that matrix in their communities. We hope that these stories resonate, inspire, and invite further conversation.

References

1. Cohn K, Friedman LH, Allyn TR. The tectonic plates are shifting: cultural change vs mural dyslexia. *Front Health Serv Manage*. 2007; **24**(1): 11–26.
2. Kirch DG. *Culture and the Courage to Change*. AAMC President's Address. Washington DC: Association of American Medical Colleges; 2007.www.ohsu.edu/xd/about/vision/upload/2007-20-AAMC-presidents-address.pdf
3. Inui T. *A Flag in the Wind: educating for professionalism in medicine*. Washington, DC: Association of American Medical Colleges; 2003.
4. Kohn L, editor; Institute of Medicine. *Academic Health Centers: leading change in the 21st century*. Washington, DC: National Academy Press; 2004.

5. Kirch DG, Grigsby RK, Zolko WW, *et al.* Reinventing the academic health center. *Acad Med.* 2005; **80**(11): 980–8.

6. Whitcomb ME. Academic health centers: sustaining the vision. *Acad Med.* 2004; **79**(11): 1015–16.

7. Bowe CM, Lahey L, Armstrong E, *et al.* Questioning the "big assumptions." Part 1: addressing personal contradictions that impede professional development. *Med Educ.* 2003; **37**(8): 715–22.

8. Bowe C, Lahey L, Kegan R, *et al.* Questioning the "big assumptions." Part II: recognizing organizational contradictions that impede institutional change. *Med Educ.* 2003; **37**(8): 723–33.

9. Scott T, Mannion R, Davies HT, *et al.* Implementing culture change in health care: theory and practice. *Int J Qual Health Care.* 2003; **15**(2): 111–18.

10. Kaldjian LC. Teaching practical wisdom in medicine through clinical judgement, goals of care, and ethical reasoning. *J Med Ethics.* 2010; **36**(9): 558–62.

11. Judge TA, Bono JE, Ilies R, *et al.* Personality and leadership: a qualitative and quantitative review. *J Appl Psychol.* 2002; **87**(4): 765–80.

12. Chervenak FA, McCullough LB. Professionalism and justice: ethical management guidelines for leaders of academic medical centers. *Acad Med.* 2002; **77**(1): 45–7.

13. Chervenak FA, McCullough LB. The moral foundation of medical leadership: the professional virtues of the physician as fiduciary of the patient. *Am J Obstet Gynecol.* 2001; **184**(5): 875–9.

14. Brater DC. Infusing professionalism into a school of medicine: perspectives from the dean. *Acad Med.* 2007; **82**(11): 1094–7.

15. Cottingham AH, Suchman AL, Litzelman DK, *et al.* Enhancing the informal curriculum of a medical school: a case study in organizational culture change. *J Gen Intern Med.* 2008; **23**(6): 715–22.

16. Ardelt M. Wisdom and life satisfaction in old age. *J Gerontol B Psychol Sci Soc Sci.* 1997; **52**(1): P15–27.

17. Ardelt M. Empirical assessment of a three-dimensional wisdom scale. *Research on Aging.* 2003; **25**(3): 275–324.

18. Branch W, Mitchell G. Wisdom in medicine. *The Pharos.* 2011; Summer: 12–17.

19. Task Force on Academic Health Centers. *Envisioning the Future of Academic Health Centers: final report of The Commonwealth Fund Task Force on Academic Health Centers.* New York, NY: The Commonwealth Fund; 2003.

20. Kohn LT, Corrigan JM, Donaldson MS, editors; Institute of Medicine. *To Err is Human: building a safer health system.* Washington, DC: National Academies Press; 1999.

21. Wachter RM. Patient safety at ten: unmistakable progress, troubling gaps. *Health Aff (Millwood).* 2010; **29**(1): 165–73.

22. Delbanco T, Bell SK. Guilty, afraid, and alone: struggling with medical error. *N Engl J Med.* 2007; **357**(17): 1682–3.

23. Wu AW. Medical error: the second victim; the doctor who makes the mistake needs help too. *BMJ.* 2000; **320**(7237): 726–7.

24. *Unmet Needs: teaching physicians to provide safe patient care; a report of the Lucian Leape Institute Roundtable on reforming medical education.* Boston, MA: National Patient Safety Foundation; 2010.

25. Bell S, Moorman D, Delbanco T. Improving the patient family and clinician experience after harmful events: the "when things go wrong" curriculum. *Acad Med.* 2010; **85**(6): 1010–16.

26. Plato. *Plato: the last days of Socrates*. Tredennick H, translator. Middlesex: Penguin Books; 1969.

27. Plato. Apology 17A, 17D–19D. In: Kaplan J, editor. *Dialogues of Plato (The Jowett Translations)*. New York, NY: Simon & Schuster; 1950.

28. Aristotle. *Metaphysics*. Ross WD, translator. Oxford: Oxford University Press; 1924.

29. Thomson, J.A.K. *The Ethics of Aristotle: the Nicomachean Ethics translated*. Baltimore, MD:Penguin Books; 1953.

30. Clayton V, Birren J. Wisdom across the life span: a re-examination of an ancient topic. In: Baltes PB, Brim OG, editors. *Life-Span Development and Behavior*. Vol 3. New York, NY: Academic Press; 1980. pp. 103–35.

31. Bluck S, Glück J. From the inside out: people's implicit theories of wisdom. In: Sternberg RJ, Jordan J, editors. *A Handbook of Wisdom: psychological perspectives*. New York, NY: Cambridge University Press; 2005. pp. 84–109.

32. Sternberg RJ. Wisdom and its relations to intelligence and creativity. In: Sternberg RJ, editor. *Wisdom: its nature, origins and development*. Cambridge: Cambridge University Press; 1990. pp. 142–60.

33. Jeste DV, Ardelt M, Blazer D, *et al*. Expert consensus on characteristics of wisdom: a Delphi method study. *Gerontologist*. 2010; **50**(5): 668–80.

34. Baltes P, Smith J. Toward a psychology of wisdom and its ontogenesis. In: Sternberg RJ, editor. *Wisdom: its nature, origins and development*. Cambridge: Cambridge University Press; 1990. pp. 87–120.

35. Baltes P, Staudinger U. Wisdom: a metaheuristic (pragmatic) to orchestrate mind and virtue toward excellence. *Am Psychol*. 2000; **55**(1): 122–36.

36. Sternberg RJ. A balance theory of wisdom. *Rev Gen Psychology*. 1998; **2**(4): 347–65.

37. Sternberg RJ. What is wisdom and how can we develop it? *Annals AAPSS*. 2004; **591**: 164–74.

38. Ardelt M. Wisdom as expert knowledge system: a critical review of a contemporary operationalization of an ancient concept. *Hum Dev*. 2004; **47**: 257–85.

39. Kinghorn W. Medical education as moral formation: an Aristotelian account of medical professionalism. *Perspectives in Biology and Medicine*. 2010; **53**(1): 87–105.

40. Ardelt M. How wise people cope with crises and obstacles in life. *ReVision*. 2005; **28**: 7–19.

41. Glück J, Bluck S, Baron J, *et al*. The wisdom of experience: autobiographical narratives across adulthood. *Int J Behav Dev*. 2005; **29**(3): 197–208.

42. Pascual-Leone J. Mental attention, consciousness, and the progressive emergence of wisdom. *J Adult Dev*. 2000; **7**(4): 241–54.

43. Tedeschi RG, Calhoun L. Posttraumatic growth: conceptual foundations and empirical evidence. *Psychol Inq*. 2004; **15**(1): 1–18.

44. Calhoun L, Tedeschi R. *Handbook of Posttraumatic Growth: research and practice*. New York, NY: Lawrence Erlbaum Associates; 2006.

45. Kleinman A. The art of medicine: a search for wisdom. *Lancet*. 2011; **5**(378): 1621–2.

46. James W. *The Varieties of Religious Experience: a study in human nature*. The Gifford Lectures Edinburgh 1902. Modern Library ed. New York, NY: Random House; 1902.

47. Plews-Ogan M, Owens JE, May NB. Wisdom through adversity: learning and growing in the wake of an error. *Patient Educ Couns*. 2013; **91**(2): 236–42.

48. May N, Plews-Ogan M. The role of talking (and keeping silent) in physician coping with medical error: a qualitative study. *Patient Educ Couns*. 2012; **88**(3): 449–54.

49. Plews-Ogan M, Owens J, May N. *Choosing Wisdom: strategies and inspiration for growing through life-changing difficulties.* West Conshohocken, PA: Templeton Press; 2012.
50. Staudinger UM, Glück J. Psychological wisdom research: commonalities and differences in a growing field. *Annu Rev Psychol.* 2011; **62**: 215–41.
51. Meacham J. The loss of wisdom. In: Sternberg R, editor. *Wisdom: its nature, origins and development.* Cambridge: Cambridge University Press; 1990. pp. 181–212.
52. Souba WW. The being of leadership. *Philos Ethics Humanit Med.* 2011; **6**: 5.
53. Souba W. Perspective: a new model of leadership performance in health care. *Acad Med.* 2011; **86**(10): 1241–52.
54. Sternberg RJ. A systems model of leadership: WICS. *Am Psychol.* 2007; **62**(1): 34–42.

Part 2

Fostering Capacities for Wisdom

THE CHAPTERS THAT FOLLOW ARE CENTERED ON FUNDAMENTAL capacities of wise leaders and the essential components of creating a wisdom atmosphere in which members of the academic health science center community can "grow up in wisdom." These capacities include finding and understanding the deeper meaning of things, reflection, compassion, understanding and applying right action in difficult circumstances, seeking out and fostering the best in ourselves and others, and understanding and embracing complexity.

Some of these chapters are preceded by an interview or a story that paints a vivid picture of the concepts discussed in the ensuing chapter. You, our readers, no doubt have your own stories of when you experienced deep meaning in your work, or compassion, a mindful moment, or an experience of bringing out the best in a colleague or a patient. You have stories of helping a colleague "do the right thing" in a difficult circumstance, a time when you "leaned into" the complexity and ambiguity of a problem and found a solution in that complexity, or a time when you noticed and valued the relational aspect of your work with good outcome. We encourage you to reflect on those stories as you read and make these chapters your own.

Fostering Meaning

WISE PERSONS SEEK TO UNDERSTAND THE DEEPER MEANING OF THINGS and events. Wise leaders seek to foster the deeper meaning and purpose in the communities they lead. Health care has deep and intrinsic meaning, yet our health-care communities struggle to stay connected to the deeper meaning of their work. In the story that follows, health-care leader Joe Mamlin tells a story that exemplifies that deep meaning in his work. He talks about this meaning as his "ultimate concern" and describes it with one word: "love." The story he tells is one of love, clinician to patients, and back around. The chapter that follows is about how leaders can connect to that deeper meaning and foster that connection in their academic health science center communities.

A Story: The Ultimate Concern

Thomas S. Inui: An Interview with Joe Mamlin

Following his internship and residency, Joe Mamlin and his wife, Sarah Ellen, spent 2 years living in Jalalabad, Afghanistan, while Joe worked with a medical school there. He subsequently helped establish the Kenya and Moi University partnership for the Indiana University School of Medicine. Joe and Sarah Ellen first lived in Kenya in the mid-1990s while Joe served as the program team leader. When they returned in 2000, they saw a country changed by the HIV epidemic and set to work to do something about it.

Now, Joe jumps out of bed every morning, ready to go and smiling.

On a beautiful afternoon in Eldoret, Kenya, Joe sat down with Tom Inui (TI), now

---

the Joe and Sarah Ellen Mamlin Professor of Global Health Research at Indiana University, to talk about finding meaning in work and in life.

TI: So, here's a different kind of a question. This is almost an impossible question, but something will pop into your mind. I'd like you to think of a time in your AMPATH work in which—and it might be yesterday or it might be in 1993—a moment, an event, a circumstance—a specific one—you felt very good about what you did. You felt effective. You felt at your best, like you really made a difference in being yourself. And then tell me the story of that event.

JM: I must be the luckiest guy in the world, because those experiences, if not daily, are weekly, year after year here, because the nature of the engagement re-expresses and affirms the meaning I found in the lifestyle that we've now made ours. It's affirmed so often and in so many different ways that I bet if I took the time, I'd find 200 of them. Obviously, they relate frequently to patients.

I'll tell you the story of one lady—her name's Jane. She was 9 months' pregnant, and she had head and neck cancer that had closed off her throat till she couldn't swallow and could not speak. And she had active herpes zoster going down her right arm so it was almost dysfunctional. I don't know if you've seen the sympathetic dystrophies that can occur when zoster . . . I always worry about it hitting an eye but now I worry about extremities. I see a lot of dysfunctional hands that are a sad consequence of that dermatome. She had an arm problem, 9 months' pregnant, and a choking cancer that was out like a bull.

Alan Rosmarin (the oncologist) was here on his first trip. I grabbed Alan and said, "What do we do?" We made a plan that we would do a tracheostomy in this woman to get control over her airway, and then induce her labor, get control of the baby—and here she's HIV positive on top of all that—and then we would try some kind of salvage chemotherapy once the baby was out and safe, and see if we could open up her airway and open up her neck. And this turned out to be a wildly malignant squamous cell carcinoma by biopsy. While we were making elaborate strategic plans, she went into labor and delivered the baby without event. So much for women's messages to well thought-out plans by doctors.

TI: And you hadn't done a tracheotomy.

JM: No, we didn't get a chance. We've all had that experience when we pull that plug and the patient keeps breathing, and the family looks at you . . .

So, I started the chemotherapy, things that I don't have a long history of doing myself. But I did with Alan's suggestion—he's long gone, so I just did it. The tumor melted, her mouth opened up and I was able to start her on antivirals. This is now a year and a half later. The baby was not infected—we were able to be so fortunate with that. And when she walks in to see me in the clinic, she always hands me the little boy and he sits in my lap and just plays with my shirt and plays with my penlight or whatever. His name is Joe Mamlin and he's the most beautiful little boy. And I hold him like our whole purpose to being here is to give birth to this little boy. I'm going to lose Mama. I know that. We can't cure this squamous cell carcinoma, but she's had a wonderful remission. And she's had a wonderful time with this child. She's totally abandoned. I pay her rent, we provide her food, and we've given her a life, and she cares in a loving way for this little boy. And then we'll see what life brings after she dies. If I were younger, he would come into our life but we're too old for that.

But I can look as I hold that little boy and maybe put a peck of a kiss on the back of his head. And just feel that life is rich, life is full. And it has nothing to do with all the things I thought one had to attain—the labels, possessions, or anything else. It's all defined in just the engagement of the moment. The now. That which expresses what everything past and future are about is experienced in the now. And those moments are powerful. And they occur frequently here.

TI: You just said something about the little boy sitting on your lap. Joe, this story is in some sense a miraculous story, and it's just a miracle that something like this can happen. It's just so improbable that something like this can happen. What is it about you as an individual that allows this miracle to unfold from an encounter in a village with a horrendous circumstance, someone so in trouble.

JM: There is a level of communication of answering questions like that at different levels. And I know fundamentally that, at the deepest level, I spent most of my life struggling through doubt and questions. I have a pretty good sense of the answer to that for myself. I'm not saying I won't say what I think, but one of the things that one learns quickly is that when things are of deep meaning to you whenever expressed in words, they look like fake jewelry. They turn to tin. They seem genuine and 24 carat when they're deep inside you, but when you use the foibles of words and so forth, and you get them out, they somehow don't quite look up to what you thought they were when they were tucked inside. And so there's a tendency for the things that are most deeply important that keep your foundation stable not to let them get too far out lest they display fewer carats than you thought. Having said that, I'm a person that is driven—at least to the extent I can be—to spend a lifetime understanding what I am really concerned about. I have tried as hard as I can to anchor myself in clarity about what my ultimate concern is. There are so many things that can compete for that anchor position in life. And without going any further than to say the answer to that question for me is *love*, period—however deeply you can take that word, and wherever you can go with it. I can say that I have to get up in the morning, have to go to bed at night driven by that ultimate concern. And that ultimate concern will condition every decision, if it's in an AMPATH board meeting, if it's at the bedside on a ward, or if it's a child sitting on my lap in clinic. To the degree that I can stay faithful to that ultimate concern, it defines my moments of meaning. It constitutes my humanity.

2

Fostering Meaning

Ann Kellams and Bryce Kellams

The alarm clock goes off at 5:45 a.m.

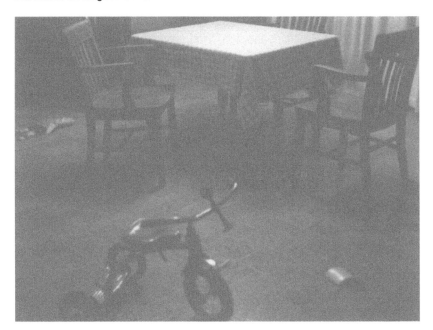

She crawls out of bed. She dresses and wakes the children, makes sure they have all the checks, signatures, snacks, and homework in their backpacks. She kisses her husband before she leaves so he knows to get up and take over.

The division meeting starts at 7 a.m. and already the 15 faces appear worn out. The division head starts in with the latest updates: we need to see more patients, a nurse triage system to help with mommy calls is tabled, we are extending our office hours, we are counting RVUs (relative value units), Dr. X is leaving as of May, Dr. Y is retiring come June, and so far we do not have any plans for replacement. There is a groan. Then, she rides the elevator up to take over the service where three new medical students, a resident on her first week of the rotation, and a nurse practitioner immediately begin to approach with nervous questions about their clinical duties, abnormal lab values, concerns about patients, and then the charge nurse with the news that we are full and really need to expedite discharges. Rounds are a blur, and she finishes just in time for her to get her food and arrive only 5 minutes late for the multidisciplinary lunch meeting, again with tired faces. Then, she gets an e-mail, one of over 200 that day, stating she and four other colleagues have received National Institutes of Health funding—almost impossible in this economic climate. Rather than joy or excitement, her first thoughts are: "Oh my, how will I fit this in? Who will cover for me? What does this mean for my family? For my division that already feels strapped? How will this be received?" She delivers the news to the chair of her department with a palpable sense of dread, concern about how this will all play out. He smiles and says, "First, congratulations! We will make this work; this is a good problem to have." He gets it. This is an honor. Patients and our department and the university will benefit. She feels relief, a hint of excitement, and a sense of renewed purpose.

This chapter addresses myriad questions about meaning in medicine and its power to change an academic health science system.[1] What defines meaning? What role does meaning play in our lives? What happens when a health system creates conditions that obscure the connection with meaning? What challenges do current conditions in academic medicine present to the meaningful practice of medicine? What happens when this connection is fostered? What is the evidence of the effect of meaning on performance, retention, satisfaction, and patient care outcomes? What practical steps can leaders in academic health science centers take to achieve excellence, and lead the change that will create a sustaining culture of meaning?

What, Then, is "Meaning" in Medicine?

Meaning is defined as import, a sense of purpose or significance.[2] Meaning, in practice, is much more than a definition. "Meaningfulness refers to the degree to which life makes emotional sense and that the demands confronted . . . are perceived as being worthy of energy investment and commitment."[3] Without meaning, we are vulnerable in the face of adversity. Dr. Rachel Remen[4] describes meaning as a human need:

> It strengthens us, not by numbing our pain or distracting us from our problems, or even by comforting us. It heals us by reminding us of our integrity, who we are, and what we stand for. It offers us a place from which to meet the challenges of life.

Viktor Frankl,[6] the physician who founded "logotherapy" (meaning therapy), cites an extreme example of the importance of meaning. While in concentration camps during World War II, he observed that only people who had a clear sense of meaning and purpose were able to overcome the extreme suffering of the camps and retain their humanity and their dignity.[5,6]

For each health-care provider, office, hospital, or health system, the meaning or significance of health care is highly individual. According to Frankl,[6] every person's meaning is unique and must be discovered, never dictated by another. Yet, all meanings are not created equal. Some meanings have the power to sustain while others have the power to destroy. The impact of meaning is crystallized by Dr. Remen's[4] retelling of the Italian psychiatrist Roberto Assagioli's[7] parable about three stonecutters working side by side on a building in the Middle Ages. The story goes that each stonecutter is apparently doing the same job, cutting rocks into blocks. Imagine approaching the first stonecutter to ask him what he is doing. He responds with irritation, "Can't you see what I'm doing? I'm cutting rocks into blocks, one after the other, all day long. It is back-breaking work, and I can't wait for each day to be over." You move quickly down the line to the next stonecutter and ask him what he is doing. "I am earning a living for my family," he says with resolve, "this is hard work, but with my skills, my children may have a better life than me." Finally, you ask a third stonecutter the same question. He looks up at you from his work, beaming, and says, "We are building a great cathedral and with the help of my skills, these walls will stand for hundreds of years to come and serve people in need of sanctuary and peace!" All of these workers are doing the exact same job, but with a clearly different sense of meaning.[4,7] Having worked in the health-care field for 20 years now, it is clear that all three of these Middle Ages mentalities are still in operation. Given the ups and downs of clinical and academic health care, individual health-care providers might even find themselves entertaining all three ways of thinking in a single day.

While it is easy for health-care providers to fall prey to the first stonecutter's experience of the routine and rigors of daily work, through its inherent values of beneficence and service, the health-care field offers a unique opportunity to achieve meaningful work.[8] There are common themes that run through those who have been called to health care. Rabow *et al.*[9] performed a qualitative analysis of the personal mission statements of medical students taking the Healer's Art course in the United States.[1] In the final exercise of this nationwide course, the students are asked to make a summary statement of their highest values of their work, the meaning of their future career. For these medical students, the most common reasons they had come to the profession of medicine were to make a difference, to connect with people in a way that is not otherwise possible, to grow as a person, and to take on a new identity as a healer in a profession of service.[9] Their study provides evidence that the meaning that calls future health-care workers to the field comes from a deeper place of personal growth and service, separate from recognition or remuneration.

Practicing physicians have also given us insight into the meaning of a health-care career. Horowitz *et al.*[10] analyzed the writings of attendees at workshops at annual meetings of the American College of Physicians and the Society of General Internal Medicine. The participants were asked to briefly write about a work-related experience that was meaningful to them. Once again, the majority of the stories involved one of three major themes: personal growth in the form of a fundamental change in perspective, a personal connection with patients, or a difference made in someone's life.[10] Dr. Remen[4] describes meaning as "the antecedent of commitment." The more meaningful our work is to us, the more invested we are in it. Reconnection with meaning in one's work can be a way to strengthen a health-care provider's motivation for and attachment to their career.[11]

What Happens When Meaning is Neglected? What is the Danger of Meaninglessness?

Just yesterday, I had dinner with a colleague in internal medicine. I asked him how things were going at his office. His response was revealing:

> OK, I guess, most days go by without much trouble, just a lot of the same interspersed with a rare disaster. I think I've finally been able to handle this computer record, but I am dreading the next EMR [electronic medical record] system we are changing to. We're supposed to be paperless, but l still can't get out from under the mountains of forms and paperwork.

I thought about my own day and, to my horror, realized that what I carry home is often that same feeling. When I am able to peel myself away from all of the electronic demands of documentation, order entry and ICD-9 codes, and find time in the room with my patients to listen, I feel good about my work. However, as soon as I leave the room, those moments are virtually washed away by the tide of paperwork, documentation, coding, meaningful use, phone messages, and lab letters. I feel as if I may never get home. By the time I leave the office, I have nearly forgotten about the kindergartener who drew me a picture, the garbage collector who had proudly lost 30 pounds by counting calories on his cell phone, and the hairdresser who shared for the first time her story about her childhood abuse.

Never has the field of health care been so rife with the opportunity for effective, coordinated, and technologically advanced services. Our continued advancement in research and development, institution of quality-of-care initiatives, emphasis on evidence-based interventions, and enhancement of data-capturing capabilities and communication strategies brought by electronic record keeping have opened the door to highly informed, consistent, and effective health care. Yet this potent change has been simultaneously coupled with the imperative to reduce health-care costs in our struggling economy. Now is the time to maximize the use of our health-care resources for the greater good of our health-care system and for our patients. While this could be good for health care, these same pressures may be, as we speak, causing significant, insidious harm to the primary source of motivation and purpose that providers carry within them, the meaning they ascribe to their work.

As we have seen in the previous section, meaning is what brings the healer back time and again, and enables them to see through the often difficult, demanding, and distracting details of a health-care system. It is the meaning in their work that keeps them going on weekends, holidays, late at night, and in bad weather. A health-care provider's sense of why they are there is what commits them to forging an honest and caring connection with a patient under any conditions. This connection is not only necessary for a patient to gain trust, but is also highly valued by the clinician. There is a positive feedback loop, and from this, a healing relationship grows. It follows, then, that anything that makes it difficult for a provider to connect with patients would jeopardize the experience of meaning and commitment as well.[9,10] Unfortunately, there are many forces at work in our current health-care climate that may do just that.

In an effort to combat the potential for errors and omissions made more common by the complexity and rapidity of our current care delivery, broad population-based and evidence-based guidelines, check lists, and other such techniques of standardization and automation are employed. The recent general acceptance of the paperless electronic medical record is aptly positioned as a tool to this end. Yet, this very strategy also often removes the individual patient from the equation and dehumanizes the interaction between doctor and patient. Providers feel like technicians and patients feel like a number. When decisions are made based on large population data and documentation done on templates, gone is the flexibility needed to respond to the nuances of the individual patient's story. This has been described as movement toward "transactional" care and away from "relational" care. This modernization of the medical care interaction "undermine(s) opportunities for ad hoc social interactions" with patients, and produces a "loss of unplanned, unscripted exam room conversations."[12] Timothy Hoff[12] describes this trend as the potential "deskilling" of a generation of physicians. We run the risk of health-care providers losing discretion, autonomy, decision-making skills, and knowledge. A provider's role as an individual may become less important and less meaningful. Running through the unrealistic and ever-growing checklist of items that must be addressed at each health-care visit in the same amount of time only adds to the anguish, as the providers feel routinely that they are not able to carry out all that they feel they should be doing.[13]

So many clinicians, ourselves included, have just recently made the transition to an EMR system and so can attest to the robust challenge that this brings. In response to the demand placed on us by the intense documentation requirements of the EMR system, we have become bogged down with finding short cuts, catchphrases, time-saving templates, and macros. So much of the time allotted for a patient visit is now spent documenting "meaningful use" of the EMR system and justifying the level of care to insurance companies, coders, and billers. Completing a note feels like working a cash register—if only the patient came with bar codes. The distracting nature of the many "point and click" programs available inevitably steals away attention and eye contact. In short, the presence, attentiveness, and spontaneity necessary for caring interactions are in jeopardy. Hoff[12] refers to the "loss of the story" to describe the "cookie cutter" interactions that are necessary to ensure that each item on the checklist is covered.

The latest movement in primary care, the "patient-centered medical home," is gaining in acceptance as well. With its goal of a comprehensive, integrated system of care brought about through the use of continuous quality improvement, electronic record keeping, physician extenders, group visits, and enhanced multidisciplinary communication, this model has the potential for increased oversight, efficiency, and the prevention of redundant care. Yet, the downside may once again be a loss of connection that doctor and patient feel when their "primary doctor" becomes a case manager of sorts. A physician who enters her or his career with the notion of service probably was not imagining punch lists and checkboxes. The types of connections the students referred to in their mission statements did not include the cables and wires on their computers.

Now combine this stress from mechanization of health care with intensified cost-containment measures. In an effort to reduce the percentage of our national gross domestic product spent on health care, Medicare and Medicaid cuts are being employed, and practices, hospitals, and particularly academic health science centers are being forced to become correspondingly more efficient. The amount of time for the health-care "transaction," then, is accordingly shorter. A provider must work either faster or longer, or both. Donelan et al.[14] referred to the "medical marketplace" in their 1997 article in *Health Affairs* and spoke of the connection to the meaning of a providers' work being stretched thinner. Greenawald and Bogdewic[15] describe the "gerbil wheel" that medical practice has become. The strongest predictors of change in a physician's satisfaction were changes in measures of clinical autonomy, including increased hours worked and the physician's ability to obtain needed services for his or her patients.[16] In essence, a doctor's satisfaction was closely tied to his or her ability to provide the quality of care that he or she felt necessary. It is easy to conclude that this is likely the case for other health-care disciplines as well. Dissatisfaction, then, is directly related to a loss of meaning: the provider does not feel he or she can provide the quality care necessary to make a difference in his or her patient's life. Landon *et al.*[17] showed, not surprisingly, that dissatisfied physicians were two to three times more likely to leave medicine. Academicians may be especially prone to burnout, as Maslach *et al.*[18] have found that both care-giving and teaching professions are among the top jobs facing attrition. For physicians, attrition may be associated with increasing levels of inefficacy, and for teachers, it may be associated with increasing levels of exhaustion.[18] In academic medicine, a loss of meaning for physicians can lead to seeking rewards in other ways, such as status, recognition, or financial gain, all of which breed competitiveness and can undermine organizational goals.[19]

Perhaps the most talked about and arguably the most severe consequence of loss of meaning for physicians is burnout. Burnout is the syndrome described by Maslach *et al.*[18] that comprises three components: (1) emotional exhaustion, (2) depersonalization, and (3) diminished feelings of personal accomplishment. It has been shown that burnout can lead to increased medical errors,[20] suboptimal patient care,[21,22] and decreased patient satisfaction.[23] Measures of burnout were also found to strongly predict career satisfaction[24] and, as mentioned earlier, the likelihood of leaving the profession.

What Happens When Connection With Meaning is Fostered? What is the Evidence of the Effect of Meaning on Clinician Performance, Retention, Satisfaction, and Patient Care Outcomes?

The University of Virginia is currently participating in a large learning collaborative with the main goal of improving maternity care and breast-feeding support in hospitals across the country. One of the steps involves placing the baby directly on the mother's chest and leaving the two of them together without separation for at least the first 1–2 hours after delivery.

This turns out to be more difficult than it sounds, as the nurses and physicians must also assess the infant, taking vital signs, performing a thorough exam, attaching the security bands and transponders, and administering the routine medications in the first few hours—all of which the nurses and physicians felt was most efficiently performed in the nursery. When the change was first discussed

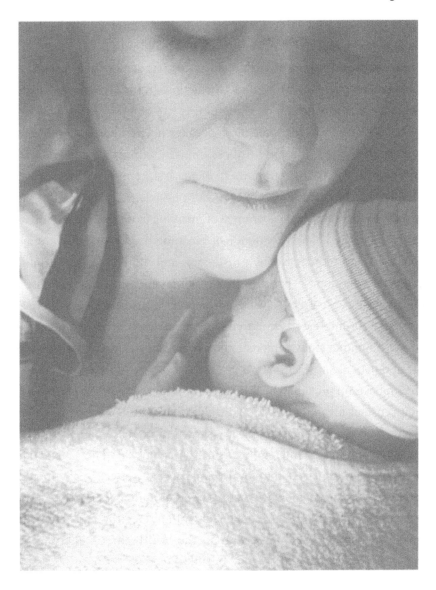

it was met with resistance. This was a common theme in the workshops at the learning collaborative. Some hospitals were further along in the implementation of this step than others. Our team heard from one hospital that had decided to roll this step out first just for vaginal deliveries a couple years ago. What began to happen as soon as they started was that there was a noticeable difference in the satisfaction of the mothers as well as the nursing and physician staff. The babies cried less and had more stable vital signs. The change really took hold when the staff was able to see and understand the real meaning of the step for mothers and their babies. Without any further mandate, the staff began to make this happen for mothers with operative deliveries on their own, and now, 2 years later, they say that no one would consider going back to the old way.

Studies in the business and health-care industries demonstrate a clear connection between employee meaning and satisfaction. In turn, employee satisfaction and empowerment, of which meaningfulness is a component, is closely correlated with performance, retention, and, perhaps most important, with customer or patient satisfaction.[25] In the business industry, an investment in loyalty and employee satisfaction has been shown to increase stock prices.[26] Workers who are satisfied tend to be more productive.[27,28] For physicians, a large part of satisfaction relates to their personal experience of meaning in their work. An investment in increasing a physician's experience of meaning has been shown to decrease burnout rates and to increase job satisfaction and fulfillment, and would likely increase staff retention.[24,28] For clinicians, studies have found that a connection to meaning is positively correlated with satisfaction.[29] Correspondingly, there is good evidence that this increased employee satisfaction leads to increased patient satisfaction.[23,30] Another study demonstrated a perfect correlation between employee morale and patient satisfaction.[31]

An emphasis on providing health-care employees with the opportunity to fulfill their sense of meaning inevitably involves pursuing quality patient-centered care. This type of care has been clearly shown to increase patient satisfaction, compliance, and both mental and physical outcomes.[32–34] The satisfaction that patients feel then translates into loyalty and reuse of services.[32,33,35] In addition, patient-centered care models with enhanced communication between health-care providers and patients have been shown to reduce the likelihood of costly malpractice litigation.[36–39] Such efforts in the health-care industry to provide patient-centered care are clearly good business.

What Practical Steps Can Leaders in Academic Health Science Centers Take to Achieve Excellence and Create a Sustaining Culture of Meaning That Will Foster Quality Patient-Centered Care? How Do We Begin to Lead This Change?

While meaning may be a human need that is essential for quality work, it does not follow that we naturally create the time and space needed for it to prosper. In fact, the opposite is generally true in health care. In an effort to juggle and balance multiple competing priorities, time for personal reflection and collegial sharing is too often jettisoned. What practical changes can leaders in academic medicine make to ensure that meaning is a priority?

Guiding Principles: Meaning Comes From Within

Enable me to keep my humility.

Help me gain patience.

Strengthen my willingness to serve others.

Show me the meaning of my work.

Enable me to be unflinching in this place between the shadow and the soul— where the tragic and the beautiful are one. To gather all my strength and all my sweetness into a healing force of truth, hope, and light. To be in solidarity with the poor, the ill, the healthy, and the wretched—of whom I am one. And above all, nurture and cultivate the poetry in my life.

Enable me to remain focused on the joy and privilege of being involved intimately with so many people in the field of service. Help me to find my way through the tougher days remembering the passion I entered medicine with.

—Medical students, Healer's Art course held in
2005, University of Virginia

Finding meaning is a discovery process; it is personal and individual, not something that can be taught or dictated.[6] There are no experts in meaning. The degree to which one is connected to the meaning of one's work may not be correlated with specialty, years of experience, or position on the pay scale. An effort should be made to remember to level the playing field in discussions related to this topic.[31] However, in order to share their personal motivations, people need to feel comfortable and safe. The leaders of change must therefore create and exemplify authenticity, transparency, mutual trust, and good citizenship. They must take on the characteristics that are desired in all employees and the organization at large.

It is important to encourage exploration of meaning at all levels, from cleaning staff to nursing and house staff, from first-year medical students to senior physician faculty. Our experience with leading group reflection on the meaning of work is profound—groups containing very diverse members can have a remarkably similar vision of the meaning of their work. Some of the strongest and most durable motivations extend beyond self, to a broader view of serving others, a greater good.[10] What brings us to medicine will sustain us.[4,6,40]

Integrating Meaning with Life Goals

Those who believe the myth of service feel that a person's value and commitment to the profession are best measured in terms of self-sacrifice. But these believers take a very short-range view. When a practitioner looks beyond immediate tasks to the tasks of a lifetime of service, he cannot fail to realize that, to serve his patients, he must care for himself.

—Rachel Naomi Remen[41]

Especially in medicine, work and life goals may be inherently contradictory. On the one hand, there is self-interest: career, self-preservation, compensation, family, and personal interests; on the other hand there is altruism: caring for and serving others.[42] Any successful initiatives meant to lead change must address both issues and must strive to help employees integrate the two principles at the individual level. In his discussion on professionalism, Kinghorn[43] describes the "moral pressure" that physicians (and other health-care providers) face. Deans can play a vital role in fostering conditions that help people make the choices that mitigate this potential for clashes between values that are humanistically and economically oriented.[19] The balance of various important life roles has also been described as a moral issue for each individual and the management of values of the institution must not be elevated above basic concerns for the individual's moral self and/or the individual's basic concerns for justice, dignity, and his or her family.[15] As Matthew Fox[44] said in *The Reinvention of Work*, life and livelihood should not be separated but should flow from the same source. Since empathy and communication are vital to patient satisfaction, it is paramount that health providers pay careful attention to striking a healthy balance between their competing interests so they may avoid burnout and be present and focused on the relationship with their patients. A professional who is able to successfully integrate his or her work life with his or her personal life will likely be more effective in the service of patients.[24] Recognizing this, efforts to promote balance should be modeled by the leaders of the system. While it is often best to emphasize positive, solution-focused discussions, it is also important to note that "organizations and the individuals in them—while wishing to be free from endless negativity—can get value from engaging openly and with reality, as suppressed negativity leads to cynicism." Treating employees "as if they are not aware of the tensions between inspiration and reality" is counterproductive. Thus, it is necessary to find a way to "engage both the inspiration towards an ideal as well as the often less-than-perfect reality of self and the organizational context in which meaning gets expressed."[45]

Carrying Good Questions

> *You can tell whether a man is clever by his answers.*
> *You can tell whether a man is wise by his questions.*
> —Naguib Mahfouz

Creating a culture that accepts the value of meaning must be carried out with a comprehensive plan that continuously asks important questions. Superficial solutions will produce superficial results.[46] Go beyond buttons, T-shirts, and posters.[8] An authentic community must be nurtured from training onward before burnout and problems exist.[47] Efforts to promote meaning, like all cultural interventions, must be ongoing to ensure that changes persist. Rather than furnishing answers or spoon-feeding employees with slogans and dogma, start a dialog by emphasizing questions. While answers can be endpoints, questions are flexible and encourage growth and adaptation in a changing environment. Carry good questions—ask them of yourself and those around you generously and listen to the responses.[48] The following questions are easily incorporated into personal or group reflective exercises. What stands in your way of providing quality care?[49] What would help you to do your job best? When are you most energized at work? When are you at your best at work or when do you feel in the "zone"? What legacy do you want to leave?[19] What is the meaning of your work? Or, from session five of the Healer's Art course for medical students, "if your work was simply a reflection of your highest values, what would it look like?"[1] Make a commitment to practice preventive care for your organization and inoculate the staff periodically with the opportunity to reflect on these questions before imbalance becomes entrenched and emergency care for an ailing system becomes necessary.

Suggested Processes

What practical steps can be taken to lead an institution-wide change that emphasizes meaning?

Explore Collective Wisdom

It is critical to ensure that vision and values are not provided only by those in positions of power but, rather, that they emerge from the collective wisdom of everyone in the organization. Leaders can provide the opportunity for their communities to "discover" that collective meaning in an intentional process.

The process begins with identifying individuals who are naturally invested in the health and progress of the institution or group. These may be the obvious leaders such as administrative heads, directing faculty, nurse managers, or there may also be others that stand out in their work. This group should reflect broad representation from all facets of the institution. They may also be individuals whose style and reputation make it apparent that they are excellent examples of meaning in practice. These people may be identified by asking employees in different departments to name those staff members who are especially inspiring in their commitment to their work.

Hold a first meeting with the identified change makers to reflect in a group format on the meaning of each individual's work. Especially effective are exercises in which members are led on a guided personal reflection, allowed time to write down their thoughts, and then encouraged to share their discoveries one by one. Consider using questions such as those found in the preceding section "Guiding Principles: Meaning Comes from Within". Ensure that meetings are inclusive; break down the silos because everyone's work in health care is interconnected.[31] Engage employees in a dialog about what makes their work meaningful for them and devote most of the time to listening.[50] Foster creativity and uniqueness in employees rather than handing down edicts.[6] Remember that identified leaders in the power structure should participate, but they are equal players, not experts in this realm. From the discussion that follows in which members share their personal wisdom, glean a common set of values that represent the mission and meaning that the group wishes to pursue and emphasize the team approach to carrying out this mission.[45]

Utilize the chosen leaders to disseminate this same type of meeting at every level and department, encouraging similar discussions in which members share their own stories of why they were called or why they came to this work, and what purpose they assign to it.[4,40,50] To model this type of collegial sharing, leaders should share their own stories as well.[8] However, if a productive sharing session is unfolding, the leaders may choose to share their vision of meaning late in the session so as not to stifle the successful dynamic. It is helpful to use motivational interviewing techniques[51] such as open-ended questions, reflective listening, and the expression of empathy. Consider also using powerful techniques such as Appreciative Inquiry (AI), as detailed in Chapter 7, to elicit the positive vision of employees.[52]

Note that most of these techniques do not involve a lot of extra time, money, or manpower. Rather, they represent a new way of thinking and being and simply underscore a certain set of priorities and values in the work. As the culture changes, talking about meaning will become routine.[19] Opportunities for the sharing of the collective wisdom of the group will abound. Begin and end even routine meetings with especially moving examples of what touched or inspired. Encourage employees to notice examples of these moments in their day-to-day work and remind them to share examples at meetings.[8]

Make Patient-Centered Meaning the Focus of All Initiatives

Because the connection to patients and the impact on their lives is so central to the meaning that providers carry, place any initiatives in the context of patient care. Lead with patient stories and relate any changes to quality patient care and safety.[12,13] Consider having a patient speak at staff meetings to underscore initiatives.[46] Schwartz Center Rounds, multidisciplinary sessions centered on specific patient case examples, is another excellent tool that is growing in popularity.[53,54] At the University of Virginia, the very first Schwartz rounds drew over 200 people to a standing-room-only crowd as a beloved surgeon described being a critically ill patient himself in our hospital. We heard not only from him but also from the nurses and doctors who cared for him. There is probably no better way to explore service and the meaning of our work than by hearing from a colleague what it felt like to be treated, visited, and helped by members of our staff. This program has been so popular that we have had to arrange for a larger venue. It is clearly fulfilling a previously unmet need.

Shifting the focus away from employee "satisfaction" per se to employee pride in providing excellent care may resonate best with the true motivations of medical professionals. Encourage an ownership attitude in your employees, one in which they take satisfaction in creating value for patients and their families.[26] A conscious shift from focusing on specific services to instead viewing the individual patient's, and his or her family's, desire for convenience, good care, and excellent health outcomes may be useful in developing strategies.[31] Concrete reminders of the institution's patient care values and intentions may also be helpful; post service-oriented messages of meaning in frequented locations.[15] Capitalize on the fact that health care is inherently meaningful, as it is about service to patients, families, and communities.[8]

Revisit Meaning

Continue to revisit meaning on a routine, regular basis. Consider leading off all meetings with "appreciative check-ins" where clinicians might share a story of something that went well in their care of a patient.[53] Provide specific and ongoing additional training opportunities such as focus groups and retreats to employees to allow for deeper reflection on meaning in medicine.[4,8–10,47,55,56] Remember to continue opening the dialog about meaning at every opportunity and with generous listening to good questions.

Conclusion

Academic health care is in a state of flux, which some may rightly consider a crisis. There are many current forces that, if left untended, are pushing this field in directions that are detrimental to both patients and caregivers. Yet, there is great hope. As Dr. Viktor Frankl[6] found, even in the most trying of times, the guiding power of meaning can prevail. While the obstacles to positive change are many and diverse, with careful attention to the meaning of our profession, we as leaders in health care have a unique opportunity to steer the health-care system toward a brighter future.

The principles and strategies that we have discussed in this chapter are a good beginning. Changing the behavior of individuals and institutions starts with ideas and solutions like these and can grow into a new way of thinking or being. With an understanding of human behavior and a commitment to actively addressing this in effective, comprehensive ways[46] we can tackle this change at both the individual and the organizational level.[18]

Fortunately, this source of strength is already within us. Consider again Dr. Remen's[4] quote from earlier in this chapter:

> It strengthens us, not by numbing our pain or distracting us from our problems, or even by comforting us. It heals us by reminding us of our integrity, who we are, and what we stand for. It offers us a place from which to meet the challenges of life.

Meaning is a natural human need that only needs the time and conditions to be remembered under the "careful concrete guidance of teachers who themselves embody these excellences."[43] Now is the time to nurture passion;[48] let the stories of meaning begin!

We'll end with a story:

It was to be a beautiful Fourth of July. My own family and everyone I knew had plans for the day. Some would go to the lake, some would spend the day at the pool, others at backyard barbecues, and later, the fireworks. Yet, I was in my white coat riding the elevator up to the eighth floor after walking into the hospital in the dark. I was feeling more than a little bit sorry for myself. A tall, well-dressed woman wearing a visitor's tag stepped onto the elevator on the second floor and stood against the opposite wall as we moved up. Her sigh told me that, like me, she would probably rather be somewhere else. We briefly exchanged sober glances, and then quietly she offered, "You pulled the short end of the stick working on the holiday, right?" I smiled, trying to pretend as if it was no concern to me, and said, "Oh well, it's OK." We rode together silently for a few more floors and then the elevator arrived at her floor with a soft "ding." As she began to step off, she turned and said, "Well, thank you. I'm glad you are here." I never saw her again, and she will never know what a gift she gave me. I was renewed with a sense of the privilege and the purpose of my job. She gave me just the dose of meaning that I needed to get through the day.

References

1. *The Healer's Art Course: overview*. Bolnas, CA: Institute for the Study of Health and Illness. Available at: www.ishiprograms.org/programs/medical-educators-students. Accessed August 14, 2012.
2. Agnes M. *Webster's New World Dictionary*. 4th ed. Cleveland, OH: Wiley Publishing; 2009.
3. Korotkov D. The sense of coherence: making sense out of chaos. In: Wong PTP, Fry P, editors. *The Human Quest for Meaning: a handbook of psychological research and clinical applications*. Mahwah, NJ: Lawrence Erlbaum Associates; 1998. pp. 51–70.
4. Remen RN. Recapturing the soul of medicine: physicians need to reclaim meaning in their working lives. *West J Med*. 2001; **174**(1): 4.
5. Klingberg H. *When Life Calls Out to Us: the love and lifework of Viktor and Elly Frankl*. New York, NY: Doubleday Books; 2001.
6. Frankl VE. *The Doctor and the Soul: from psychotherapy to logotherapy*. 2nd ed. New York, NY: Vintage; 1986.
7. Assagioli R. Cheerfulness: a psychosynthetic technique. *Psychosynthesis Research Foundation*. 1973; **33**: 12–21.
8. Morrison EE, Burke GC 3rd, Greene L. Meaning in motivation: does your organization need an inner life? *J Health Hum Services Admin*. 2007; **30**(1): 98–115.
9. Rabow MW, Wrubel J, Remen RN. Promise of professionalism: personal mission statements among a national cohort of medical students. *Ann Fam Med*. 2009; **7**(4): 336–42.
10. Horowitz CR, Suchman AL, Branch WT, *et al*. What do doctors find meaningful about their work? *Ann Intern Med*. 2003; **138**(9): 772–5.
11. May DR, Gilson RL, Harter LM. The psychological conditions of meaningfulness, safety and availability and the engagement of the human spirit at work. *J Occup Organ Psychol*. 2004; **77**(1): 11–37.
12. Hoff TJ. The physician as worker: what it means and why now? *Health Care Manage Rev*. 2001; **26**(4): 53–70.
13. Zuger A. Dissatisfaction with medical practice. *N Engl J Med*. 2004; **350**(1): 69–75.
14. Donelan K, Blendon RJ, Lundberg GD, *et al*. The new medical marketplace: physicians' views. *Health Aff (Millwood)*. 1997; **16**(5): 139–48.
15. Greenawald M, Bogdewic S. Rejuvenate your practice. *Contemp Peds*. 2011; May: 54–7.
16. Landon BE, Reschovsky J, Blumenthal D. Changes in career satisfaction among primary care and specialist physicians, 1997–2001. *JAMA*. 2003; **289**(4): 442–9.
17. Landon BE, Reschovsky JD, Pham HH, *et al*. Leaving medicine: the consequences of physician dissatisfaction. *Med Care*. 2006; **44**(3): 234–42.
18. Maslach C, Schaufeli WB, Leiter MP. Job burnout. *Annu Rev Psychol*. 2001; **52**: 397–422.
19. Lieff SJ. Perspective: The missing link in academic career planning and development: pursuit of meaningful and aligned work. *Acad Med*. 2009; **84**(10): 1383–8.
20. West CP, Huschka MM, Novotny PJ, *et al*. Association of perceived medical errors with resident distress and empathy: a prospective longitudinal study. *JAMA*. 2006; **296**(9): 1071–8.
21. Shanafelt TD, Bradley KA, Wipf JE, *et al*. Burnout and self-reported patient care in an internal medicine residency program. *Ann Intern Med*. 2002; **136**(5): 358–67.

22. Spickard A Jr, Gabbe SG, Christensen JF. Mid-career burnout in generalist and specialist physicians. *JAMA*. 2002; **288**(12): 1447–50.
23. Haas JS, Cook EF, Puopolo AL, *et al*. Is the professional satisfaction of general internists associated with patient satisfaction? *J Gen Int Med*. 2000; **15**(2): 122–8.
24. Keeton K, Fenner DE, Johnson TR, *et al*. Predictors of physician career satisfaction, work-life balance, and burnout. *Obstet Gynecol*. 2007; **109**(4): 949–55.
25. Yukl G, Becker W. Effective empowerment in organizations. *Org Manage J*. 2006; **3**(3): 210–31.
26. Heskett JL, Sasser EW, Wheeler J. *The Ownership Quotient: putting the service profit chain to work for unbeatable competitive advantage*. Boston, MA: Harvard Business Press; 2008.
27. Baruch-Feldman C, Brondolo E, Ben-Dayan D, *et al*. Sources of social support and burnout, job satisfaction, and productivity. *J Occup Health Psychol*. 2002; **7**(1): 84–93.
28. Lin CP. Modeling corporate citizenship, organizational trust, and work engagement based on attachment theory. *J Bus Ethics*. 2010; **94**: 517–31.
29. Geller G, Bernhardt BA, Carrese J, *et al*. What do clinicians derive from partnering with their patients? A reliable and valid measure of "personal meaning in patient care". *Patient Educ Couns*. 2008; **72**(2): 293–300.
30. Atkins PM, Marshall BS, Javalgi RG. Happy employees lead to loyal patients. Survey of nurses and patients shows a strong link between employee satisfaction and patient loyalty. *J Health Care Mark*. 1996; **16**(4): 14–23.
31. Clark PA, Wolosin RJ, Gavran G. Customer convergence: patients, physicians, and employees share in the experience and evaluation of healthcare quality. *Health Mark Q*. 2006; **23**(3): 79–99.
32. Clark PA, Drain M, Malone MP. *Return on Investment in Satisfaction Measurement and Improvement*. South Bend, IN: Press Ganey Associates; 2005.
33. Stewart MA. Effective physician-patient communication and health outcomes: a review. *CMAJ*. 1995; **152**(9): 1423–33.
34. Stewart M, Brown JB, Donner A, *et al*. The impact of patient-centered care on outcomes. *J Fam Pract*. 2000; **49**(9): 796–804.
35. Kaplan SH, Greenfield S, Gandek B, *et al*. Characteristics of physicians with participatory decision-making styles. *Ann Int Med*. 1996; **124**(5): 497–504.
36. Beckman HB, Markakis KM, Suchman AL, *et al*. The doctor-patient relationship and malpractice: lessons from plaintiff depositions. *Arch Intern Med*. 1994; **154**(12): 1365–70.
37. Entman SS, Glass, CA, Hickson GB, *et al*. The relationship between malpractice claims history and subsequent obstetric care. *JAMA*. 1994: **272**(20): 1588–91.
38. Lester GW, Smith SG. Listening and talking to patients: a remedy for malpractice suits? *West J Med*. 1993; **158**(3): 268–72.
39. Levinson W, Roter DL, Mullooly JP, *et al*. The relationship with malpractice claims among primary care physicians and surgeons. *JAMA*. 1997; **277**(7): 553–9.
40. Fillion L, Dupuis R, Tremblay I, *et al*. Enhancing meaning in palliative care practice: a meaning-centered intervention to promote job satisfaction. *J Palliat Support Care*. 2006; **4**(4): 333–44.
41. Remen N. The myth of service. *New Physician*. May 1997; p. 3.
42. Jonsen A. *Clinical Ethics: a practical approach to ethical decisions in clinical medicine*. 7th ed. New York, NY: McGraw Hill Medical; 2010.

43. Kinghorn WA. Medical education as moral formation: an Aristotelian account of medical professionalsim. *Perpect Biol Med*. 2010; **53**(1): 87–105.

44. Fox M. *The Reinvention of Work: a new vision of livelihood for our time*. New York, NY: Harper Collins; 1994.

45. Lips-Wiersma M, Morris L. Discriminating between 'meaningful work' and the 'management of meaning'. *J Bus Ethics*. 2009; **88**(3): 491–511.

46. Grenny J, Maxfield, Shimberg A. How to 10x your influence. *Vital Smarts*. 2008: 1–10.

47. Rabow MW, Wrubel J, Remen RN. Authentic community as an educational strategy for advancing professionalism: a national evaluation of the Healer's Art course. *J Gen Int Med*. 2007; **22**(10): 1422–8.

48. Chapman AB, Guay-Woodford LM. Nurturing passion in a time of academic climate change: the modern-day challenge of junior faculty development. *Clin J Am Soc Nephrology*. 2008; **3**(6): 1878–83.

49. Remen RN. The recovery of the sacred. *Context*. 1994; **39**: 28–31.

50. Atchison TA. Exposing the myths of employee satisfaction. *Healthc Exec*. 2003; **18**(3): 20–21.

51. Madigan MM. Reclaiming the connectedness of medicine. *Adv Mind Body Med*. 1999; **15**(2): 136–8.

52. Hettema J, Steele J, Miller WR. Motivational interviewing. *Annu Rev Clin Psychol*. 2005; 1: 91–111.

53. May N, Becker D, Frankel R, *et al. Appreciative Inquiry in Healthcare: positive questions to bring out the best*. Brunswick, OH: Crown Custom Publishing; 2011.

54. www.theschwartzcenter.org

55. Brown S, Gunderman RB. Viewpoint: enhancing the professional fulfillment of physicians. *Acad Med*. 2006; **81**(6): 577–82.

56. Dunn PM, Arnetz BB, Christensen JF, *et al*. Meeting the imperative to improve physician well-being: assessment of an innovative program. *J Gen Intern Med*. 2007; **22**(11): 1544–52.

Fostering Reflection

THE CAPACITY FOR REFLECTION AND ATTENTION IS AN ESSENTIAL component of wisdom practice since it allows a person to go beyond self-interest and to reach outside an individual perspective to reflect on thoughts and behaviors. Cultivating this capacity guards against making the same mistake twice and being a slave to one's own way of seeing things and one's own emotions. It helps us to notice the subtleties in a patient's history, the fleeting physical finding, the change in a patient's face that signals anxiety. It is critical for benefitting and growing from life experiences. That said, fostering this capacity in ourselves as leaders and in the communities we lead is far from easy. As Schorling and Goodman point out in this chapter, fostering this reflective capacity is more a discipline than a decision, a discipline in which both leader and whole communities can engage.

3

Promoting Reflection

John Schorling and Matthew Goodman

By three methods we may learn wisdom: First, by reflection, which is noblest; Second, by imitation, which is easiest; and third by experience, which is the bitterest.

—Confucius

TOM IS A 50-YEAR-OLD PHYSICIAN AT AN ACADEMIC MEDICAL CENTER. He is highly successful, a full professor with a National Institutes of Health (NIH)-funded research program and an international reputation in his field. With the flattening of the NIH budget, he is finding it harder to maintain his funding, and his stress level begins to increase, affecting both his work satisfaction and home life. Several of his employees complain about his outbursts of anger. At the suggestion of a colleague, he enrolls in an 8-week mindfulness course. Following the course, he writes the following e-mail to his dean:

> I did take part in the Mindfulness Seminar. This was an incredibly valuable experience. The mental and physical health assessments done at the start of the session (questionnaire-based instruments) put me in the lowest third or quartile, which was also a concerning revelation. However, by the end of the program, I felt much better and this was reflected objectively in marked improvements in both assessment tools. Since then, I feel much more productive and effective, and markedly happier with work and life. I am also sure that

I am a better colleague, mentor, and friend. Though it wasn't fun to go through this, the result has been one of the most valuable growth experiences in my life, and for that I am deeply grateful.

Being a leader in health care is a daunting challenge in these times of mounting costs and declining reimbursement. These pressures are magnified in many academic health centers also faced with declining research funding as the NIH budget remains flat. Although sometimes overshadowed by these financial issues, it is crucial to remember that the role of health care is to care for patients. How can leaders of today's academic health centers address all these issues while also educating the next generation of physicians? As noted in Chapter 10, Wiley Souba,[1] vice president for health affairs and dean of the Dartmouth School of Medicine, has recently argued that the key is for leaders to focus on the "being of leadership," that leaders need to "spend much more time leading themselves." He suggests there are four foundational pillars of being a leader: (1) awareness, (2) commitment, (3) integrity, and (4) authenticity. This chapter primarily addresses fostering awareness, focusing on techniques for "revealing the hidden and unchallenged assumptions, beliefs and frames of reference that comprise our worldview."[1] In other words, in order for leaders to lead themselves, they must first know themselves.

As has been accepted since ancient times, knowing oneself is not easy. "Know thyself" was an inscription on the Temple of Apollo at Delphi, and Plato refers to Socrates using this phrase in his teachings. In particular, Socrates states that it is important that he know himself first and that until he does, "it seems to me ridiculous, when I do not know that, to investigate irrelevant things."[2] From a more contemporary perspective, in his book *The Happiness Hypothesis*, Jonathan Haidt[3] uses a metaphor of a rider on an elephant to describe the mind and the challenge of knowing oneself. The rider represents conscious, verbal thinking, which is often considered to be the whole mind, yet most of what goes on in the mind is outside of this realm and is relatively automatic, as represented by the elephant. Although the rider may think he controls the elephant, actually the elephant can wander off and do as she pleases anytime she wants. For Haidt,[3] "knowing thyself" in large part means getting to know the elephant and improving our ability to influence her.

Another way this association has been conceptualized is through emotional intelligence. Although traditional measures of intelligence are often considered to be the most important factors leading to success, including for leaders, Daniel Goleman[4] demonstrated almost 15 years ago that emotional intelligence (emotional quotient) was more important than intelligence quotient. A useful model of emotional intelligence includes four basic competencies: (1) self-awareness, (2) self-regulation, (3) social awareness, and (4) relationship management. The most important of these competencies is self-awareness.[4,5]

So how can self-awareness be cultivated in order to foster the ability to "be" a successful leader? Reflective practices can help those practices that focus on reflecting on important personal experiences and questions. A key factor relates to the rider and the elephant—if much of what the elephant does is automatic, how can we discover what the elephant is likely to do in different situations? For instance, there may be a certain type of situation in which we feel uncomfortable and tend to react in a certain way, perhaps when someone criticizes us when we do not feel it is warranted. This may result in our feeling upset and saying something we wish we had not. In this situation, we are reacting to a stimulus, often without thinking, without engaging the rider. Why is this so? Often we do not take the time to consider this question. Rather, we may move immediately to projection and justification, coming up with all the reasons why the other person was wrong and it was OK for us to respond the way we did ("that person's an idiot), or we may move to judgment, especially judging ourselves ("I must be a bad person because no good person would have yelled like that"). Yet, there is a very powerful alternative, an alternative based on openness and curiosity, that of simply noticing our reaction, without judgment, and being open to wondering why we reacted the way we did. Once we begin to be aware of our experience as it is occurring we may have the space to make a different decision, to respond rather than simply react, to engage the rider, not simply follow the elephant wherever she may go. When this happens, the range of choices we have begins to expand.

As was noted in Chapter 1, self-awareness is necessary for the cultivation of wisdom. In Ardelt's 3-D model of wisdom, one of the principal components is reflective, which includes the capacities for self-examination, self-awareness, and self-insight. According to Ardelt,[6] "only after the transcendence of one's subjectivity and projections is a deeper understanding of life possible."

Self-Assessment Tools

There are a wide variety of forms of self-examination that can increase one's self-awareness and self-insight in domains related to leadership. Standardized assessments can be very useful in increasing awareness about our preferences and behavioral tendencies, aspects of ourselves that we often take for granted, and we may even assume that others must have the same viewpoints we do. The University of Virginia has had an ongoing leadership training program since 2004 for faculty and administrators from across the university, including physicians and medical center employees. This program, called Leadership in Academic Matters (LAM), enrolls two cohorts a year of 30 participants who meet for 3½ hours once a week for 14 weeks. A major focus of this program is to foster self-awareness, including using self-assessments addressing a number of different domains. The following possible assessments do not make an exhaustive list but they cover a wide range of leadership issues. The first assessment that participants in this course complete is the Myers-Briggs Type Indicator[7] This is an assessment of personality type, and it is often the first time individuals are exposed to their own preferences and how they differ from others. Professional burnout is measured with the Maslach Burnout Inventory, which assesses burnout in three domains: (1) emotional exhaustion, (2) depersonalization, and (3) personal accomplishment.[8] As in other settings, physicians and other health-care providers in this program tend to have high levels of personal accomplishment, even if they are emotionally exhausted and are feeling depersonalized. Conflict management style is assessed with the Thomas Kilmann Conflict Mode Instrument,[9] and team participation is assessed with the Belbin Self-Perception Inventory.[10] In addition to these self-assessments, LAM program participants also have others complete 360-degree evaluations of emotional intelligence using the Emotional and Social Competence Inventory.[11] Together these assessments provide participants with a rich snapshot of their own behaviors and preferences, and this often leads not only to increased self-awareness but also to a greater understanding of important factors affecting interpersonal relationships.

Self-assessments such as these can provide important insights into why we do some of the things we do, but they are for the most part descriptive, helping to illuminate what we do, even when we may not be aware of our tendencies to act and react in certain ways. However, they often do not help us understand why we do the things we do. This usually requires a deeper level of reflection that we classify into three main practices, all of which we utilize in LAM: (1) reflective writing, (2) personal disclosure, and (3) mindfulness/awareness of the present moment.

Reflective Writing

It has been said that we write to learn what we didn't know we knew. Writing can be used in a variety of formats to increase self-awareness and well-being. In *The 7 Habits of Highly Effective People*, Stephen Covey[12] notes the importance of "beginning with the end in mind," of writing about what one wants one's life to have accomplished in order to be certain that we are headed in the right direction with our lives and our careers. As he notes, "if the ladder is not leaning against the right wall, every step we take only gets us to the wrong place faster."[12]

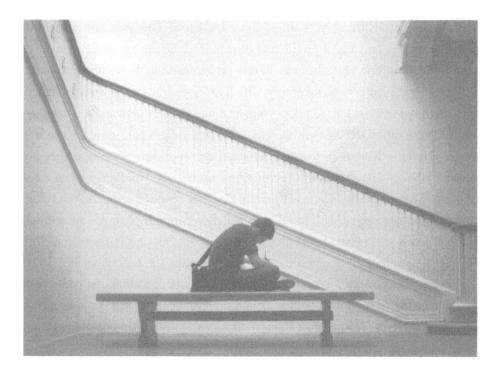

Expressive writing that includes writing about the emotional content of experiences—rather than writing only about events themselves or not writing at all—has been shown to improve well-being. James Pennebaker[13] has been studying the impact of writing on physical and psychological health since the 1980s. He notes that expressive writing is a process of labeling and acknowledging emotions, which in turn can lead individuals to interpret their circumstances differently.[13] A meta-analysis of 146 randomized trials of such disclosure found overall improvements in physiological health, physical health and overall functioning among those who practiced expressive writing.[14] Such writing helps individuals interpret and make sense of life events and to find meaning in them.[15]

A simple writing exercise that has been shown to improve well-being and decrease depressive symptoms is to write down three good things that happen each day and why. Individuals who do this for 1 week have higher levels of happiness and fewer depressive symptoms for up to 6 months.[16]

Personal Disclosure

Personal disclosure to others can be a very powerful technique to better understand ourselves. For this to be most effective, trust between individuals or within a group must be cultivated. Ground rules, including confidentiality and the freedom to speak only as much as one is comfortable, can help foster trust. Generous listening by others is also very important to making this process most productive—a prop such as a "talking stick" can be used to facilitate this, so that only the individual holding the stick speaks. Focusing on speaking from one's own experience is also important. As health-care providers we often want to give advice, yet in truly listening to others what often serves best is simply bearing witness without trying to fix anyone or anything.

There are several exercises that we have found particularly useful in helping individuals discover more about themselves. *Stepping Stones* is one. This is a process in which participants sit in a circle in a group of six to eight. Each takes a number of stones from a basket in the middle of the circle and then, taking turns, each participant uses the stones one at a time to describe events that have brought them to their current circumstance. Often participants are quite surprised by what they choose to share as seminal events in their lives. The stones serve as what Parker Palmer[17] has termed a "third thing" between the individual and his or her story that often brings out unexpected insights.

Another very powerful exercise developed by Rachel Remen[18] is "Exploring Meaning through Symbolic Objects." In this exercise, participants bring an object that will fit in their hand that represents or symbolizes the meaning of their work.

Sitting in circles of eight to ten, they then describe to others in the group the meaning of the object to them. Each person speaks about his or her object in turn, and during this process no one else in the group speaks. After each person has spoken about the object, the objects are slowly passed around so each person holds each object from their group, taking time in silence to appreciate the wisdom in it. Once the objects have been passed around the circle the groups can then ask questions of one another and discuss the process. This is often perceived by participants as the most powerful of all the sessions in the University of Virginia's LAM program, and they often comment on how much they learned about the meaning of their work for themselves, and also how much they appreciate the commitment of others to their work. As an example of an object that was shared, an anesthesiologist brought in a bird's nest, saying that she viewed her work caring for patients during surgery like that of birds caring for their eggs and their young in the nest, vulnerable and dependent.

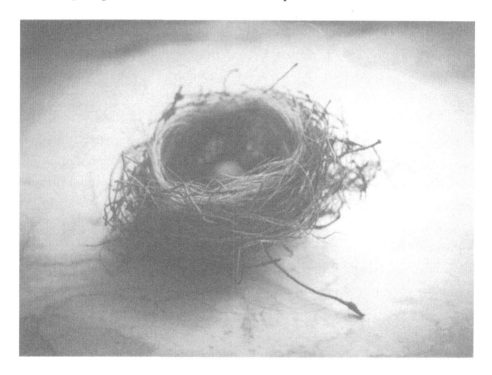

Appreciative interviews are another means of fostering self-disclosure. Appreciative interviews are used in the organizational change process based on Appreciative Inquiry (*see* Chapter 7), and involve asking questions about times when we are at our best. We often use these interviews in groups and ask individuals to pair with someone they do not know well. They are then provided a scripted question to ask each other about a peak experience. The range of potential topics is quite broad and an interdisciplinary group from the University of Virginia has published a book that contains over 75 suggestions.[19] An example of such an appreciative interview prompt is "Think about your unique gifts, abilities, and strengths as a leader. Please tell me the story of a time when you were at your best as a leader. What unique leadership gifts, abilities, and strengths did you display?" Speaking about a peak experience also often helps individuals reconnect with the meaning of their work, and to recognize more explicitly what they find most important and rewarding. Joining in "improbable pairs" and sharing a peak experience with someone from a different background or work area also often leads to a greater appreciation for the contributions of others.

A fourth, very powerful, and more in-depth self-disclosure exercise is to create and discuss family genograms to explore family of origin issues.[20] In medicine we come face to face every day with difficult situations, some of which cause strong reactions that we may not understand, or even be aware that not everyone has. Often these are based on family-of-origin issues, especially when someone violates a rule that we learned growing up. For instance, if someone grows up in a family where hard work and accomplishment are always expected, even if this is not explicitly stated, then patients who are perceived as not trying to achieve or help themselves may be viewed negatively and perhaps demeaned or blamed for their situation. Making this more apparent and recognizing that this response comes from a rule that not everyone holds to can be very helpful in understanding otherwise unconscious reactions. In doing this work, physicians who exhibit disruptive behavior are often surprised at the close correlation between their family-of-origin rules and the situations that get them into difficulty. The purpose of this exercise is not to delve deeply into where these rules originated or why they result in certain reactions when violated, but rather to recognize that these associations exist so when they come up the individual has a choice about how to respond.

Mindfulness

Practicing paying attention to our own experience is a third reflective practice that can foster "being" a leader.[21] A story of two young fish swimming together helps illustrate this. An older fish swims by and asks, "Hey boys, how's the water?" One of the young fish looks at the other and replies, "What's water?" Like the young fish, we are often unaware of our own milieu. In our case it is often the internal world of thoughts, judgments, and perceptions to which we remain oblivious.

In order to be aware of what is going on around and within us, we must first learn to pay attention, and attention is a scare commodity these days. In Kurt Vonnegut's[22] dystopian short story *Harrison Bergeron*, all people are required by law to be equal. One of the main characters, of higher than average intelligence, is rendered average by a device that distracts him with a loud buzzing noise every few minutes. In the era of pagers, beepers, and cell phones most of us now carry with us a device or two of that nature, whether by choice or as part of our professional responsibility.

In order to see ourselves and others more clearly, we can commit to a path of personal development that involves enhancing our ability to pay attention, both inside ourselves and to what is happening around us.[23] Most of the world's great wisdom traditions incorporate prayer, reflection, silence, meditation, and instructions on disciplining the attention. The practice of mindfulness—purposeful, nonjudgmental, present-moment awareness—resonates with the reflective teachings of the great religions of the world. It is possible to bring attention to our present-moment experience at any time by paying attention to thoughts, emotions, and bodily sensations as they arise. This ability to be mindful can be cultivated through formal meditation practices, such as focusing attention on breathing or parts of the body, walking meditation, and movement practices like yoga and tai chi.

At the University of Virginia we teach mindfulness as a secular discipline as part of the LAM program and also in a dedicated 8-week course for health-care providers based on the Mindfulness-Based Stress Reduction course developed by Jon Kabat-Zinn[24] and Saki Santorelli[25] at the University of Massachusetts Medical School. Course participants are introduced to body and breath awareness practices and are encouraged to bring present-moment awareness to everyday personal and professional experience. During the weekly class sessions, they share with the group their observations regarding their formal meditation practices, and bringing mindful awareness to moments of daily living.

We see measurable changes in the health-care providers who take our classes, in the form of improved mental health scores on the SF-12, and decreased levels of burnout as measured by the Maslach Burnout Inventory.[26] Researchers from the University of Rochester have also demonstrated similar effects that have persisted for over a year after completing a course in mindful communication for primary care physicians.[27] Many participants describe the University of Virginia course as profoundly moving, or life-changing. While it is difficult to reduce or fully characterize the experience of participants, over the 10 years of teaching the course we have noticed the recurrence of certain themes, several of which we will review here.

Compassion

The quality of bringing kind attention and understanding to the suffering of another along with the desire to relieve it, compassion is central to health care and institutional leadership relationships. Compassion and empathy are the topics of Chapter 5. Mindfulness, nonjudgmental present-moment awareness, is crucial to the development and maintenance of compassionate relationships.

The health-care providers who take our classes are committed professionals, and most were drawn to the field by a love of the caretaker role, and by a sincere desire to help others. What is perhaps surprising is that in this idealistic crowd we often find a profound lack of self-compassion. Compulsive traits are rampant, and overly harsh self-critical thoughts often come to light when they slow down enough to pay attention to their inner life.

Self-criticism, perfectionism, and harsh self-judgment create the conditions for dysphoria, depression, and burnout. They also undermine the ability to have authentic compassionate relationships with others. Compassion is one element of the reflective component of wisdom. Having compassion for others is important for leaders in health care who want to foster healthy work and educational environments where patients receive optimal care and students, staff, and faculty can all flourish. However, true compassion for others must be based on compassion for self. Nonjudgmental awareness of our own self-critical natures can lead to a softening of these tendencies, which makes it easier to sit in the presence of others who are struggling or in pain, without having our own buttons pushed.

Empathy

Empathy is the ability to understand another person's experience and to pay attention and respond to his or her emotions.[28] Empathy is an essential element of quality medical care, and is necessary for optimal interpersonal relationships.

A key component of empathy is self-awareness. This is necessary to recognize behaviors in others as expressions of their emotional states, and to make the distinction between the emotions of others and those of ourselves. An empathic response involves a partial identification of the observer with the other. Paying attention to one's own emotional response as it is arising in relationship with another person can facilitate this identification with the other. When we sit with someone who is experiencing a difficulty we can notice our own emotional responses, and by paying attention to them respond appropriately and authentically. Even though we may have never been through exactly the same situation or faced the identical challenge, being open to our own experience allows us to "touch in" to our own emotions, knowing that what arises in us is likely related to what is arising in our patients, our coworkers, and those we supervise. Knowing this can allow us to respond in ways that increase our connectedness and improve our relationships.

Closing off these emotional connections with others may be associated with burnout and a loss of empathy. This can result from feeling overwhelmed by the number of emotions that can arise in taking care of patients and dealing with others, especially if we feel that we have to fix what is causing their difficulties. However, often just recognizing these emotions, acknowledging them, and being present with them is enough. Mindful awareness can help us recognize when the urge to fix others' emotions arises and perhaps to let it go, focusing on what is within our sphere of influence, our own emotions and responses.

Appreciation

Thich Nhat Hanh, the noted Vietnamese Buddhist teacher, tells us that having a toothache enlightens us as to how wonderful it is not to have a toothache. The secret, he tells us, is to appreciate our non-toothache![29] In paying attention to the present moment, we can see what we are happy about and thankful for. We can feel OK about our own fine qualities and deeds, rather than feeling a need to play them down out of shame, or to exaggerate them to fill an inner void.

In health-care relationships, appreciation means that we can focus on what is right with our patients as well as what is wrong with them. We can enjoy our warm feelings toward them and their expressions of gratitude without having to diminish them or brush them aside.

From an institutional leadership perspective, we can appreciate and promote what is going right, rather than always tending to focus on what is wrong and needs to be fixed. We can even initiate a formal Appreciative Inquiry process within out institution as described in Chapter 7.

Equanimity

Eating a sandwich outdoors at a meditation retreat, a young man was bothered by a bee. He tried to wave it away, but it became more agitated and buzzed louder. This went on for several minutes, until the bee flew over to a young nun at the next table. She did not react, and the bee quickly moved away.

We can spend a lot of time and emotional energy "waving at bees" in our personal and professional lives. Mindfulness and meditation can help us to remain calm and avoid snap judgments and premature reactions to novel stimuli. The thought stream that arises in a difficult situation can be observed and evaluated rather than being taken as the truth. "Don't believe everything you think" reads the bumper sticker given to one of us by a course participant.

In our work environments, there are a great many things about which we can worry. Some of these we have some control over, and many of them we do not. Noticing our thoughts and what we are paying attention to can be very helpful in differentiating whether the thinking we are doing is likely to be productive or whether we are just spinning our wheels, wasting precious psychic energy in the process. Covey[12] refers to this issue as the choice between focusing on the large "circle of concern" of all the things we can be concerned with or on the much smaller "circle of influence" representing only those things we can actually influence. Another way of stating this is the Serenity Prayer: "Grant me the serenity to accept the things I can not change, the courage to change the things I can, and the wisdom to know the difference."

Joy

Our work is important and often difficult. We are responsible for making decisions that impact lives and careers. Our mistakes can be costly to patients, institutions, and professional reputations. All of this can feel rather heavy; it can make us walk with our heads down and our brows furrowed.

Awareness and self-compassion can soften our worried and self-critical natures a bit; allow us to unfurrow the brow and look up. We can feel the simple joy in our relationships with patients, coworkers, family and friends; enjoy the freshness of children and the beauty available in the natural world.

Don't Miss Anything

"Don't miss anything" says the intern to herself,
as she pores over the data from her most recent admission.
"Don't miss the coin lesion on the Xray,
the low potassium, the subtle anion gap.
Don't miss the eosinophilia, the macrocytosis, the mild lymphopenia."
Her list goes on.

I agree, and would like her to expand the list:
"Don't miss the patient's grateful smile when she is met with concern,
or the sudden chill in the air when talk of her child's illness
is curtailed to move on to the review of systems."

"Don't miss the warm smile of the housekeeper who greets you as you pass.
As you walk outside, don't miss the way the wind is twisting the oak leaves,
the way it feels on your face.
When you get home, don't miss the wetness of your dog's nose on your hand,
or the warmth of your child's arms around your neck."

Don't miss anything.

—Matt Goodman

Insight
· · · · · · · · · ·

Whether it is through writing, personal disclosure, or mindfulness, all of these reflective practices can foster new insights. When we slow down and take time to reflect we can gain a greater understanding of our own experiences as well as those of others and we may begin to see things in new ways. By writing, we may be better able to understand life events, through disclosure we can foster deeper connections with others and see relationships in new ways, and through mindfulness we can become more aware of our present moment experience and see how many more choices we have than we previously realized. While engaged in any of these practices, ideas that are seemingly entirely new to us may suddenly appear in our awareness, as if someone has turned on a light. Paying attention to these new insights can help us expand the range of what we consider possible and perhaps help foster greater wisdom.

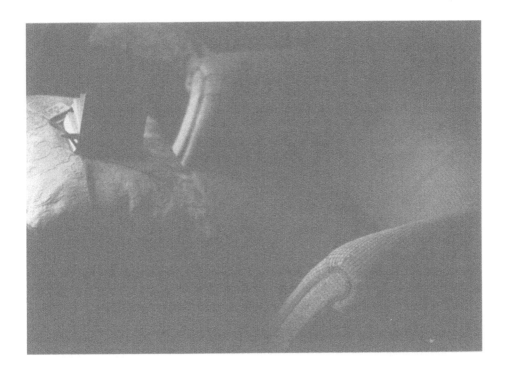

Summary

Reflective practices can help improve our self-awareness and shed light on how our predispositions and biases shape our thoughts, emotions, and behaviors. Lack of self-awareness can lead us to being consigned to simply following the movements of "the elephant" we happen to be riding, reacting to changes in direction without necessarily understanding them. Cultivating greater awareness through self-assessment tools and through reflective practices—including writing, personal disclosure, and present-moment awareness—can greatly increase the range of choices we consider in any circumstance. They can help us "be" more effective and wise leaders and can improve our quality of life in measurable ways. It is appealing to believe that promoting these practices in our institutions will nurture the idealistic professional qualities that drew many of us toward a career in health care, and keep us aligned with our deepest core values.

References

1. Souba WW. The being of leadership. *Philos Ethics Humanit Med.* 2011; **6**: 5–16.
2. Plato. *Phaedrus.* Plato in Twelve Volumes. Vol. 9. Fowler HN, translator. Cambridge, MA: Harvard University Press; London: William Heinemann; 1925. Available at: www.perseus.tufts.edu/hopper/text?doc=Perseus%3Atext%3A1999.01.0174%3Atext%3DPhaedrus%3Asection%3D230a (accessed March 18, 2012).
3. Haidt J. *The Happiness Hypothesis.* New York, NY: Basic Books; 2006.
4. Goleman D. What makes a leader? *Harv Bus Rev.* 1998; **76**(6): 93–102.
5. Goleman D, Boyatzis R, McKee A. *Primal Leadership.* Boston, MA: Harvard Business School Press; 2002.
6. Ardelt M. Wisdom as expert knowledge system: a critical review of a contemporary operationalization of an ancient concept. *Hum Dev.* 2004; **47**: 257–85.
7. Hirsh SK, Kummerow JM. *Introduction to Type in Organizations.* Mountain View, CA: CPP; 1998.
8. Maslach C, Jackson SE, Leiter MP. *Maslach Burnout Inventory Manual.* 3rd ed. Palo Alto, CA: CPP; 1996.
9. Thomas KW, Kilmann RH. *Thomas-Kilmann Conflict Mode Instrument.* Mountain View, CA: CPP; 2007.
10. *Method, Reliability & Validity, Statistics & Research: a comprehensive review of Belbin team roles.* Belbin; 2013. Cambridge, England. Available at: www.belbin.com/content/page/5835/BELBIN(uk)-2013-A%20Comprehensive%20Review.pdf (accessed July 11, 2013).
11. *Emotional and Social Competency Inventory.* Hay Group. Available at: www.haygroup.com/leadershipandtalentondemand/ourproducts/item_details.aspx?itemid=58&type=1&t=2 (accessed July 11, 2013).
12. Covey SR. *The 7 Habits of Highly Effective People.* New York, NY: The Free Press; 1989.
13. Pennebaker JW, Chung CK. Expressive writing, emotional upheavals and health. In: Friedman H, Silver R, editors. *Foundations of Health Psychology.* New York, NY: Oxford University Press; 2007. pp 263–84.
14. Frattaroli J. Experimental self-disclosure and its moderators: a meta-analysis. *Psychol Bull.* 2006; **132**(6): 823–65.
15. Wilson TD. *Redirect.* New York, NY: Little, Brown & Company; 2011.
16. Seligman MEP, Steen TA, Park N, *et al.* Positive psychology progress: empirical validation of interventions. *Am Psychol.* 2005; **60**(5): 410–21.
17. Palmer PJ. *A Hidden Wholeness: the journey toward an undivided life.* San Francisco, CA: John Wiley & Sons; 2004.
18. Remen R. *Exploring Meaning with Symbolic Objects.* Bolnas, CA: Institute for the Study of Health and Illness; 2007.
19. May N, Becker D, Frankel R, *et al. Appreciative Inquiry in Healthcare: positive questions to bring out the best.* Brunswick, OH: Crown Custom Publishing; 2011.
20. Nichols MP, Schwartz RC. *Family Therapy: concepts and methods.* Needham Heights, MA: Allyn & Bacon; 2001.
21. Epstein RM. Mindful practice. *JAMA.* 1999; **282**(9): 833–9.
22. Vonnegut K. *Welcome to the Monkey House.* New York, NY: Dial Press; 1998.
23. Boyatzis R, McKee A. *Resonant Leadership.* Boston, MA: Harvard Business School Press; 2005.

24. Kabat-Zinn J. *Full Catastrophe Living: using the wisdom of your body and mind to face stress, pain, and illness.* New York, NY: Bantam/Dell; 1990.
25. Santorelli S. *Heal Thy Self.* New York, NY: Bell Tower; 1999.
26. Goodman M, Schorling JB. A mindfulness course decreases burnout and improves well-being among healthcare providers. *Int J Psychiatry Med.* 2012; **43**(2): 119–28.
27. Krasner MS, Epstein RM, Beckman H, *et al.* Association of an educational program in mindful communication with burnout, empathy, and attitudes among primary care physicians. *JAMA.* 2009; **302**(12): 1284–93.
28. Neumann M, Bensing J, Mercer S, *et al.* Analyzing the "nature" and "specific effectiveness" of clinical empathy: a theoretical overview and contribution towards a theory-based research agenda. *Patient Educ Couns.* 2009; **74**(3): 339–46.
29. Hanh, Thich Nhat. *Peace Is Every Step: the Path of Mindfulness in Everyday Life.* New York, NY: Bantam Books; 1992.

Supporting Humility, Forgiveness, and Trust

ONE POWERFUL OPPORTUNITY FOR THE DEVELOPMENT OF WISDOM IS a situation of adversity or moral conflict, critical situations where our deepest selves are challenged. One could surmise that how we treat those situations in our academic health science center both reflects and determines our growth in wisdom as individuals and as a community. These "critical situations" in health care include when things go wrong, when we are stressed, when we are morally challenged, and circumstances of conflict. As a leader, paying attention to how we frame and respond to these situations as a community may be key opportunities for fostering wisdom, in our trainees, in ourselves, and even in our patients.

The story that follows is one leader's personal response to a major medical error at her hospital, her reflection on the deeper values that stood behind her response, and her own growth in its wake. The subsequent chapter centers on the concept of professionalism and tells the story of how one organization has created a matrix in which these difficult and challenging critical situations can be approached with an intent to foster learning, trust, growth, and wisdom.

A Story: When Things Get Tough

Ora Hirsch Pescovitz

When I was CEO at Riley Hospital for Children in Indianapolis, I had personal experience with a serious medical error. One night, when I was the administrator on call, I had a chilling experience that forever changed my approach to patient safety.

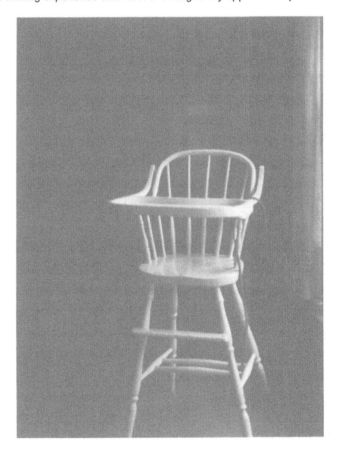

My husband, Mark, and I were at a black-tie event when my BlackBerry buzzed. The message said: CALL—EMERGENCY. I learned that five vulnerable premature babies in the NICU (neonatal intensive care unit) in Methodist Hospital had received a terrible overdose—adult dosages of heparin, a blood-thinner to prevent clotting. The drug's manufacturer had streamlined packaging to simplify its use, but this caused confusion as to which vials contained adult doses and which contained the much smaller pediatric doses.

I left my husband at the concert and told him to find his own way home, and I rushed to Methodist. On the way, I called the NICU and learned that medication to counteract the heparin had already been given without any noticeable improvement. I knew that meant the situation was terribly serious. I contacted Sam, the system's chief operating officer, and Linda, the chief nursing officer, who were attending another black-tie event and I told them to meet me at the hospital. Within minutes, the three of us arrived on the unit—all of us dressed in formal evening wear. That alone signaled to staff who saw us running into the hospital that something was terribly wrong. I entered the NICU. The unit was nearly full of babies—26 of them, with only one crib unused. Babies were crying. Frantic parents were crying. One mother demanded the names and addresses of specific nurses and vowed revenge on those she believed were in the process of killing her infant. No, I thought, that's not what happened. This was a medical error, a very serious error, the most serious one I had ever seen. Questions had to be answered: What exactly had happened? Who was involved? Where were they? How would order and control be restored? What was the best path to care for the affected babies and others in the unit? What about the families?

And, what should I do? Though it was late Saturday night, I called additional neonatology staff at home and asked them to please come in to assist with the crisis. They did so willingly. I spoke with the many chaplains who had arrived to provide support and comfort, and I helped direct them to the frightened and grieving parents and terrified staff. In addition, I asked for a summary of events from the unit's nurse practitioner and neonatologist. After reviewing the number of adult heparin vials that were missing, contemplating the chaos of the situation and hearing the reports, I had a sudden realization that there must have been a sixth baby who was given a heparin overdose. During the next several minutes, we identified a sixth baby. Care to this child was initiated immediately.

After 6 long and grueling hours in the NICU, I finally got to my car and started it. That was the moment when the tears just flowed; I allowed myself to feel the tragedy at an emotional level—before that point, I could not break down. What good would that emoting have done when there was so much work to do? Alone in my car, I allowed my own vulnerabilities to be exposed. I had never seen anything like what I had just witnessed.

In the end, two babies died within the first 24 hours and a third baby died a few days later; three babies lived, including the sixth one we had identified. The entire institution was changed in perpetuity as a result of this calamity. I was forever changed. Patient safety became the mantra across every unit in the system and I was reminded why it is so important to never be content and to always be improving. No matter how good we think we are, we can always be better. This is fundamental to my leadership philosophy.

One of the most powerful lessons I learned that day was about the real meaning of leadership. I think that Donald McGannon (a devoted advocate of broadcasting's potential for good) summed it up best when he said that "Leadership is action, not position." In the moment, I somehow knew what to do and how to act. It just fell into place naturally for the three of us—Sam, Linda, and me. Somehow we knew how to make order out of chaos in an environment that felt like a war-zone. In the follow-up analysis—looking at how something like this could happen and getting to the root cause—I learned valuable lessons, which I've applied since at the University of Michigan. What it comes down to is that health care is a human system, and humans are fallible. There is not and never will be a perfect physician or nurse, or a perfect hospital. The most educated, experienced, and well-intended people make mistakes, and the most prestigious health care organizations make medical errors. That is why a culture of safety requires processes and systems that minimize human error and a culture with a zero tolerance policy for blame.

There are other people in the story. Teams contribute to any and all successes. You may hear about certain "rock stars," but make no mistake, there are teams behind them. Personally and professionally, we are strengthened by others, and we grow and evolve by being open to and learning from diverse perspectives.

Atul Gawande said, "There is . . . a central truth about medicine . . . all doctors make terrible mistakes. The important question isn't how to keep bad physicians from harming patients; it's how to keep good physicians from harming patients." Like me, all health care professionals have to learn to get comfortable with the uncomfortable so that, eventually, we can serve others and provide them with comfort. As my own career has evolved, I am no longer merely comfortable with discomfort, I now embrace it, because I have concluded that it is actually this discomfort that leads us to strive to learn more, to discover more, to do more, to work harder, and ultimately to do it better.

Those of us who work in health care are truly among the most fortunate in the world, because people place their trust in us during their most vulnerable moments. Nothing is more powerful, and no responsibility is greater. Health care culture is very complex—especially in an academic medical center, which brings together learners, medical professionals, scientists, and administrative and operations employees from diverse backgrounds and specialties. You can have academic traditionalists working with tech-savvy Millennials, administrators sharing space with entrepreneurs, history experts partnering with visionaries. I think that this is terrific, because these intersections are where ideas are conceived and innovation is born. All of this change pushes me to continuously learn and develop as a leader, so that I understand the challenges, changes and trends that impact the organization and so that I am evolving as well. I love the energy of an academic medical center environment because of this!

As a health care leader, to make sense of this and to lead within this complex and multicultural environment, you stay true to your values in everything you do and every decision you make. And, you take time to learn from every interaction. I abide by what essayist Robert Greenleaf called "servant leadership." I regard my primary role as a leader to be creating environments in which others can thrive. I know I am never the smartest person in the room—I am there to learn and get smarter just like everyone else. I like to surround myself with diverse perspectives and even contradicting opinions. I encourage my team to take risks when it makes sense, to embrace failure as opportunity and to be nimble in response to change. Academic medicine and health care are constantly evolving and changing in response to the evolving and changing needs of patients, scientific discoveries and the sociopolitical climate. With health care issues taking center stage in the current political environment, we know that unprecedented changes are ahead, so it is incumbent upon us to be ready for that and all change, and, in fact, to lead.

I would also say that an example of relational social sciences is the work I am doing with my leadership team. We are working with a coach to improve how we interact and function. Until you have full trust among members, you won't have a team that is maximally successful and productive. Teams go through phases. They morph and change as the environment changes and as new people come on board. There is even the question of what "the team" is and who should be part of it. As a physician-scientist, I learned the importance of learning through observation; of remaining objective and letting experiments—not preconceived notions—reveal the truth. As a hospital administrator, I've learned how important it is to be a member of a productive team. And as a mother of three, I learned that my role was creating a nurturing, comfortable environment from which my children could emerge to be maximally successful. My leadership style is a culmination of all of these experiences and this combination helps me balance authority and intimacy, logic and emotion. Wisdom comes from active listening, humble self-awareness, and lifelong learning. These qualities can certainly promote the type of health care culture that succeeds and leads, remains nimble and progressive, and embraces the continuous improvement of its practices and people.

4

Supporting Professionalism and Trust

Jo Shapiro and Sara Nadelman

Professionalism and Its Definitions: Spectrum and Similarities

How an organization or institution defines professionalism or professional behavior depends on the culture, the leadership and the broader expectations of the profession. Medicine has extensive definitions, publications, and academic theories about professionalism. But beyond the platitudes and definitions, what does professionalism really mean and how do we foster it in the academic medical center?

In medicine, some of the most commonly referenced standards for professionalism include those from the Accreditation Council for Graduate Medical Education (ACGME), the Association of American Medical Colleges, and the American Board of Internal Medicine. The American Board of Internal Medicine's[1] *Medical Professionalism in the New Millennium: A Physician Charter* delineates principles and commitments to being a professional physician. The ACGME's *Common Program Requirements* lists commitment, adherence, and sensitivity as the three prime components of postgraduate medical professionalism.[2] Other institutions, such as Virginia Commonwealth University, have created a standard of conduct for all students and faculty that include honesty, maintaining confidentiality, respect, and ethical behavior.[3] The University of

Kansas University Medical Center lists specific components of professionalism including altruism, accountability, excellence, respect for others, and a personal commitment to lifelong learning, duty, honor, and integrity.[4]

Swick[5] asserts that medical professionalism

> consists of those behaviors by which we—as physicians—demonstrate that we are worthy of the trust bestowed upon us by our patients and the public, because we are working for the patients' and the public's good. Failure to demonstrate that we deserve that trust will result in its loss, and, hence, loss of medicine's status as a profession.

The Association of American Medical Colleges'[6] *Assessment of Professionalism Project* gives a framework for developing and evaluating professionalism in medical schools through a multilateral approach to teaching and assessment. These documents touch on communication, transparency, honesty, and forthrightness in all interactions. In medical education circles, the Flexner Report[7] and its updates are seen as the seminal overview of professionalism in medical schools. The Liaison Committee on Medical Education, the ACGME, the Joint Commission, and other medical oversight bodies cite professionalism as competencies in medical education and development.[8] These documents make recommendations regarding behavior and ethical practice but cannot provide the day-to-day oversight required for culture change. At our institution, we define professionalism as anything that builds trustworthy relationships. Highly professional behavior engenders honest, empathic relationships and is inextricably linked to providing safe, high-quality patient care.

This chapter will outline one reproducible multifaceted approach to culture change and professionalism in the academic health science center (AHSC): the Center for Professionalism and Peer Support (CPPS) at Brigham and Women's Hospital (BWH).

A New Definition of Professionalism

Our definition of professionalism—*anything that builds trustworthy relationships*—can be applied to both work and life environments. Professionalism creates an environment that promotes respectful communication at all levels.

This communication can change the culture of health-care institutions and is directly tied to patient safety and optimal patient care.[9] The CPPS's specific focus is the physician's relationship to the health-care team, but it also includes clinician–patient relationships as well as scientists' interactions with their teams.

Professional Identity

During the developmental process of becoming a clinician, students look for leaders, mentors, supporters, and colleagues from whom they can learn to develop their professional identity. Getting mixed messages and interpreting them through a lens of the oft-repeated platitude of "professionalism" can be confusing and difficult to navigate during all stages of development. Finding a way to teach professionalism to all physicians in a humane, realistic, non-punitive fashion to all physicians remains a challenge. Medical students are often "taught" professionalism via lectures. Follow-up is sparse, often only occurring if there is a breach of conduct serious enough to trigger being called into the dean's office. Reinforcement of good professional behavior is often lacking. Therefore, students bring their individual interpretation of professionalism into their internship experience, probably one of the most challenging years of their training. Throughout their residency and fellowship programs, trainees, amidst the myriad responsibilities and expectations levied on them, are expected to embody professionalism at all times or risk reprimand. Having strong, compassionate role models and support structures in place for these trainees is necessary for them to have the foundation to continue building their professional identity and demeanor.

How does one even begin creating a culture change that helps engender professionalism? While there is no clear algorithm, we believe that the process should be intentional and multifaceted, requiring the buy-in of institutional leadership, practitioners, and team members. There are few institutions that have taken on this task explicitly. What follows is a narrative about the complexities of leading an organizational change effort to foster professionalism by creating a community of support and an atmosphere of honesty, trust, and continuous learning. This story of how the BWH's CPPS came into being shines a light on how incremental change can make a difference in the culture and the definition of culture at an academic health center. The CPPS teaches professionalism, handles professionalism lapses, and provides various forms of peer support, disclosure and apology coaching, wellness programming, educational offerings on giving feedback and difficult conversations, and other programs tailored to the needs of clinicians and scientists.[10]

Professionalism and Culture Change

Many of us have become increasingly aware of a loss of a sense of community and support at our AHSCs—faculty, trainees, and students are experiencing more and more pressures and demands with less and less sense of shared purpose and support. The BWH has a highly skilled group of clinicians, scientists, and health-care team members who care deeply about their work, including clinical care, education, and research. And yet we feel the pressures of increased clinical demands, higher patient expectations, less research funding, and little support for teaching. Appropriately, there is a focus on improving patient care, meeting credentialing mandates, getting more funding, and continuing to meet the increasing credentialing requirements for training programs. Yet, at certain moments, such as after adverse events or malpractice claims, we tend to withdraw support from one another. How can we expect those who are feeling overwhelmed, vulnerable, and afraid to be able to deliver high-quality compassionate care? It was with this in mind that we created the Center to focus on high standards of interpersonal relationships and explicit support during difficult times.

We have unique leadership at BWH. In particular, Anthony Whittemore, MD (the former chief medical officer [CMO]), with the support of Gary Gottlieb, MD (the former president), put some resources into developing programs that were beginning to address some of these issues. Some of the nascent programs included professionalism training sessions for all of the physicians, a group peer support program, and a defendant support group. We then decided to pull these programs under one umbrella and expand and develop each in the context of the others.

The first thing we did was to bring together a group of trusted advisors. We formed a community of people across our institution with unique and valuable perspectives on leading change. Some of these people also were leaders of groups with whom we wanted to partner, such as risk management, credentialing, employee assistance program, patient family relations, the office of general counsel, and so forth. This kind of work should be done "in community," with a true sense of shared responsibility. These concepts are taught by facilitators and colleagues in Leading Organizations to Health, a professional development group based on the principles of relationship-centered leadership. In addition, we began by building on the strengths and resources already in place at BWH. Loosely based in the Appreciative Inquiry approach (as discussed in Chapter 7), we took the already-established programs and began to slowly grow and expand their scope and depth. For example, we were learning a great deal about the perceptions of professionalism from the rich discussions during the professionalism training sessions. In addition, we collected data from the anonymous Behavior at Work Surveys that we administered during the sessions. This led us eventually to rewrite the professionalism training materials.

The concept of emergence, one of the principles of adaptive complex systems (which will be discussed in Chapter 8), was helpful in framing our approach. A good example of this was the addition of a 1:1 peer support program that we developed in parallel to the established group peer support program. We found that the group peer support was immensely helpful to most of the health-care team members who had been affected by an emotionally stressful event such an unanticipated patient outcome or the death of a colleague. However, the affected physicians did not tend to participate in such sessions, or if they participated, it was in the role of team leader rather than a colleague in need of support. We also conducted a study that showed physicians would strongly prefer having a colleague provide support after an adverse event. Therefore, we designed an innovative system using trained physician peer supporters to reach out to affected physicians after an adverse event or lawsuit. We have expanded this training to nursing as well.

One of the most important principles has been using a multifactorial approach to the complex adaptive challenges we are tackling. The most powerful illustration of this is the professionalism initiative. Dr. Anthony Whittemore[16] had years ago recognized the need for institution-wide education regarding professionalism, and he developed a training program in partnership with a group of employment law educators. In creating the CPPS, we realized that in parallel to this educational initiative there needed to be a robust hearing concerns program to deal with the lapses in professionalism exhibited by any member of our institutional community. While individual hospital leaders will choose various ways to lead their institutional culture initiatives, lessons learned in creating the BWH's CPPS can be translated to a variety of situations that change leaders might find useful in their own development of professionalism and peer support programs. There is no culture manual for institutions. We make our own culture and can change the culture on both a micro and a macro level each day.[11]

Hearing Concerns Program: Dealing with Disruptive Physicians

In order to retain credibility in our commitment to supporting a culture of mutual respect throughout the institution, we need to hold everyone to the same high standards of respectful behavior. The Center provides a safe place for anyone to voice concerns regarding unprofessional behavior they have witnessed or experienced on the part of any BWH physician. This includes an assessment process as well as partnering with the physician's supervisory physician to discuss a remediation and follow-up plan. Such a process needs to be backed by strong leadership. We received that support with Gary Gottlieb, MD, and we continue to receive it with Betsy Nabel, MD, the hospital president.

The definition of disruption/disruptors is broad: anything or anyone that potentially disrupts communication either within the health-care team or between the patient and the health-care team. The Joint Commission cites disruptive behavior as having a direct link to poor patient safety outcomes.[9,12–17] Disruption often occurs as the interplay between personal accountability and systems issues. Disruptors tend to see themselves as staunch patient advocates and those who do not stand with them as people who are not as committed to patient care as they. Their disruption has likely worked in the past and, as a result, disruptors prioritize their needs above others. Often disruptors don't realize the gap between their intended results such as improved patient care, and their impact, such as team demoralization and the resulting patient safety risks. The CPPS faculty has these difficult conversations with disruptors. The disruptor should be offered resources that might help them gain insight into the impact of their behavior, such as 360-degree evaluations, coaching, communication training, and so forth. The disruptor then has to make a decision if he or she wants to change or not. You cannot force behavior change, but you can enforce consequences.

The "hearing concerns" program allows anyone in the hospital to come to the CPPS director or associate director in a confidential manner to discuss their concerns about physician professionalism. Over the 4 years this program has existed, there have been approximately 170 full investigations. An investigation involves an initial complaint where someone comes forward with professionalism concerns regarding a physician or scientist. The CPPS then asks for others whom they might contact to find out more regarding the person about whom concerns were raised (the "focus person"). The CPPS director then meets with the others who were named by the contact person (the initial person who raised the professionalism concern), without identifying this initial person, and discusses the focus person further. The next step involves bringing this multisourced data to the focus person's supervisory physician and coming up with a plan. Using her experience in dealing with professionalism lapses, the CPPS director serves as a coach or advisor to the supervisory physician in how to approach the disruptor.

In any major culture change effort, there are likely to be perceived and sometimes real challenges to the status quo. The strongest example of this was in the handling concerns program. In centralizing this process, we anticipated that some clinical leaders might feel that we are encouraging people to "go behind their back" or air their departmental or divisional dirty laundry in a more institutionally public way. We decided to address these concerns directly during formal and informal conversations with chairs and chiefs. As Ron Heifitz and Martin Linsky[18] point out, one of the jobs of a leader is to acknowledge what will be lost in the change. Our program does involve some perceived loss of autonomy on the part of the clinical leaders, so we felt this should be acknowledged and discussed. We frame this as a true partnership: we can only accomplish our shared goals— delivering the highest-quality patient care, research, and education—together.

Framing the initiative as a patient safety issue was the most powerful impetus to achieve buy-in from all of our leaders. One year after the CPPS started, the Joint Commission delivered its national mandate for a zero tolerance policy for disruptive behaviors.[9] This was helpful in underscoring our institution's message: the quality of care delivered and taught, scientific discoveries made, and workplace productivity is dependent upon the establishment of and continued nurturing of respectful relationships throughout our entire institution.

One of the keys to the success of this program is that the CPPS has the support of the hospital president, CMO, and key hospital leaders, including the department chairs. If it is determined that a disruptor has not changed his or her behavior in a reasonable amount of time, he or she may be asked to leave. Over the past 3 years 10–12 people have left the institution based almost solely on professionalism issues. This is not a number that the CPPS relishes, but it does show the institutional community that unprofessional behavior will not be tolerated, even if it means losing an influential, financially productive practitioner. The vast majority have instead chosen to change their behavior so that they can continue to be a part of our institution. It has been said that people cannot change their character but they can change their behavior.

Peer Support: The True Peer Model

It is intuitively clear that being in a supportive environment is likely to facilitate professional behavior. Conversely, if a clinician feels afraid, ashamed, and judged, he or she may be at risk for unprofessional behavior. Causing harm to a patient is one of the most challenging moments of a physician's career. A clinician who has been involved in an error resulting in harm to a patient may feel highly vulnerable, both emotionally and socially. Although we know that most adverse events involve systems errors, not personal shortcomings, there is an appropriate sense of personal responsibility that clinicians should and do feel after an error. Often this sense of personal responsibility leads to a sense of despair.

Making an error can be devastating for a physician. Many physicians experience significant emotional and job-related stress following serious errors and near misses. According to a 2007 study through the Washington University School of Medicine, of 3171 physicians in the United States and Canada surveyed after an adverse event, 61% experienced increased anxiety about future errors, 44% experienced a loss of confidence, 42% experienced sleeping difficulties and reduced job satisfaction, and 13% felt the event harmed their reputation. The study reported that physicians' job-related stress increased when they had been involved with a serious error. In addition, one-third of physicians involved in near misses also reported increased stress. Only 10% agreed that health-care organizations adequately supported them in coping with error-related stress.[19] It is clear that physicians need support, although their likelihood of seeking it remains low. In a recently published study, physicians stated that they would most like support from other physicians after an adverse event. However, they do experience several barriers to seeking such support.[20] What is the best approach to providing peer support to a group that generally doesn't seek out this kind of resource?

The referrals for peer support often come from risk management but can also be requested by colleagues or the clinicians themselves who are directly involved. The peer supporters do not provide counseling, but they refer to counseling services or other resources as necessary. The program is focused on being contacted by a supportive colleague who understands what they are going through. This is a unique model as it is focused on and targeted to physicians and nurses who may otherwise not be willing to actively seek support. The peer support interventions are kept strictly confidential. In addition to the one-to-one peer support model, the CPPS offers group peer support to teams who have been involved in a stressful event. Employee assistance program leaders run these programs, and everyone on the team who has been affected by the event is invited to attend. This group support can be repeated over time as needed by the team. In addition, we have a discrete defendant support program for any clinician named in a lawsuit. This includes both a letter from the CPPS director and CMO to the defendant expressing support as well as contact information for several physicians who have been sued and are available to answer questions and provide support.

The aim of these programs is not to remove the clinician's emotions following an adverse event—these emotions are normal and come from a place of caring and personal responsibility. Rather, we hope to facilitate resilience so that the clinician goes beyond recovery and on to learning and wisdom. In the best circumstances, the clinician will experience personal growth and will help his or her colleagues make systems changes to prevent the adverse event from occurring in the future. Attaining such resilience and wisdom can best happen in a just culture where support is a given.

Disclosure and Apology

The disclosure and apology movement in medicine, with its pioneering researcher Dr. Thomas Gallagher from the University of Washington, has opened the door for an honest discussion of how we interact with patients after an adverse event or a near miss.[21-23] Learning how to provide transparent communication with patients after an adverse event or near miss is a vital tool in the professionalism kit. Even those who have practice delivering bad news do not do it often enough to be left without supports before and after the disclosure. The Center has set up a disclosure and apology-coaching program where trained disclosure coaches are available 24 hours a day, 7 days a week and can advise clinicians on how to disclose and apologize to the patient and family. Rehearsing the specifics of what the attending physician will say is crucial to his or her preparation for what is always a difficult process. At the same time, the clinicians have a peer supporter to help them manage their own emotions.

Professionalism and Leadership

Developing as a leader is a lifelong process of increasing self-awareness and relational skills. Programs that teach relationship-centered leadership, leadership development, organizational change management, mindfulness, and gaining wisdom can all contribute to one's growth as a leader. One powerful professional development group that facilitates leadership in health care is Leading Organizations to Health.[24] The teaching in Leading Organizations to Health is based on the work of Parker Palmer, an educator and activist. He emphasizes self-knowledge, attunement to the group, development of communication, and

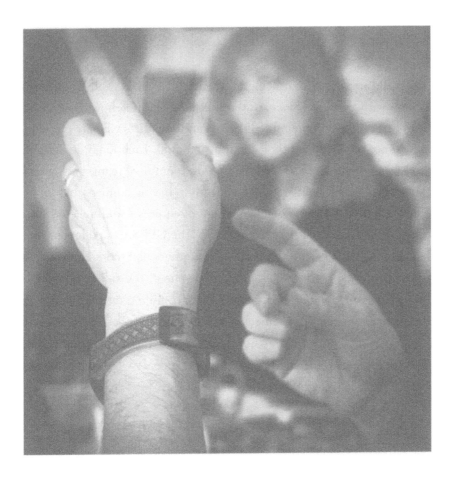

relationship-centered leadership. The experiential learning promotes building deep community connections and leveraging group wisdom. The work is rooted in organizational change theory and science. It is important that such leadership development includes applying theory to actual practical organizational leadership challenges.

Another way to support leadership development is to find mentors and sponsors. Mentors are those who provide guidance and leadership as you develop your physician identity. Sponsors are people in leadership positions who are well established in the field and who will put you forward for opportunities that arise. They push you to take on new roles and become known in your field via speaking engagements, conference attendance, and the like. The most important aspect of mentors or sponsors is that they are right for you and your path. These relationships change over time and you will need different mentors/sponsors for your different professional roles and education.

Lessons for Organizational Program Development

The Center did not come into being overnight. There was, and is, an ongoing conversation with thought leaders in the hospital regarding how to support the BWH's professional environment. Clinicians and scientists who are emotionally depleted cannot work toward their highest potential. Emotional depletion can be caused by such stressors as working in a dysfunctional team, having experienced an adverse event, being named in a lawsuit, having family issues, or being chronically fatigued. A professionalism program requires a multifaceted system. The approach we took to garnering support for the CPPS was collaborative and included genuine inquiry into those areas that others had more knowledge and experience with. Recognizing that autonomy is one of the values prized by the clinicians, scientists, and administrative staff is an important part of success.[25] Organizational change has to balance autonomy with the good of the institution and those it serves. Understanding how to balance opposing viewpoints, needs, and priorities gives you a frame for working with people who might not understand your mission or may have competing priorities.

Choosing a Champion for Developing Professionalism Programs

The lead person needs to be someone who is respected not only by their peers but also by all levels of teams and staff with whom they work. No one is perfect, and it is wise for any professionalism leader to admit to his or her own shortcomings. Having leadership education and a strong self-awareness would be an important asset. Since AHSCs face mounting financial responsibilities and productivity goals, being given the time or resources to start a professionalism program may be difficult. Ideally, having a full-time professionalism leader who has appropriate administrative support would move the mission forward more quickly, but with commitment to culture change, institutional support, and a strong proposal you will be able to slowly build a sustainable professionalism program. A proposal should include a mission statement outlining the general goals of the program and a detailed explanation of the different elements. As the program grows and develops, you will need the latitude to make changes and mold it to the institution's needs.

This is a story of how one of our Center's programs might foster a clinician's capacities of self-reflection, right action, and humility.

Sam Smith, MD, is a mid-career academic internist. One of his patients has just had an adverse event leading to harm, including a serious infection and a prolonged hospital stay. The complexities of the case are such that at first no one knows exactly why this happened. After further review, it is apparent to Dr. Smith that the patient did not receive the appropriate antibiotic for the infection. Only Dr. Smith and the resident know about this. If they said nothing, the patient would not have any way of knowing that there was an error. Dr. Smith is devastated. He prides himself on his clinical skills, including an excellent fund of knowledge and compassionate care. He feels sad for his patient as well as guilty and ashamed. He knows that if he tells the patient about the error, he places himself at risk for being sued. In addition, his reputation as an expert clinician may suffer. He is having difficulty sleeping at night and he cannot concentrate well at work. Fortunately, he knows about the disclosure and apology and peer support programs. He calls a peer supporter, and they have an in-depth open conversation where Dr. Smith shares his concerns. During this intervention, the peer supporter has helped Dr. Smith put this event in the context of his many years of practice and excellent outcomes.

They talk about personal responsibility as well as systems changes needed to help naturally occurring medical errors from reaching a patient. They talk about how our culture sometimes views medical errors as moral failings rather than as the result of our being human and working in complex systems. Dr. Smith recognizes that his perfectionism, which often serves his work well, can now be a source of boundless self-recrimination that may interfere with his emotional healing. Dr. Smith decides to call risk management and a disclosure coach who can help him disclose and apologize to the patient in a way that is transparent and empathic, as difficult as this is, given how awful Dr. Smith feels about what has happened. Upon Dr. Smith's alerting the CPPS, the resident receives an outreach peer support call. In addition, Dr. Smith includes the resident in the disclosure and apology conversation with the patient so she can observe and learn.

Given the incredible complexity as well as deep responsibility of our work, we know that we will each experience significant stressors in the course of our professional and personal lives. It is our moral responsibility as institutional leaders to help create a community that fosters trust and respect of the individuals and teams that provide the clinical care, research and teaching that make AHSCs so valuable. No one program or center can accomplish this imperative, but leaders at AHSCs can think about ways they can lead change, even in the face of monumental challenges.

References

1. American Board of Internal Medicine (ABIM) Foundation. *Medical Professionalism in the New Millennium: a physician charter.* Philadelphia, PA: ABIM Foundation; 2002 [cited January 3, 2013]. Available at: www.abimfoundation.org/Professionalism/Physician-Charter.aspx
2. Accreditation Council for Graduate Medical Education (ACGME). *Professionalism Explanation.* Chicago, IL: ACGME; 2008 [cited January 3, 2013]. Available at: www.acgme.org/acgmeweb/Portals/0/PDFs/commonguide/IVA5e_EducationalProgram_ACGMECompetencies_Professionalism_Explanation.pdf
3. Professionalism Committee of the School of Medicine. *Professionalism Committee Report.* Richmond, VA: Virginia Commonwealth University School of Medicine; 2001 [cited January 3, 2013]. Available at: www.medschool.vcu.edu/professionalism/standards/documents/vcusom_professionalism_cmte_report0901.pdf
4. University of Kansas School of Medicine. *Professionalism Initiative.* Kansas City, KS:

University of Kansas Medical Center; 2013 [cited January 3, 2013]. Available at: www. kumc.edu/school-of-medicine/pdfa/profesionalism-initiative.html

5. Swick HM. Toward a normative definition of medical professionalism. *Acad Med*. 2000; **75**(6): 612–16.

6. Association of American Medical Colleges. *Assessment of Professionalism Project*. Washington, DC: Association of American Medical Colleges; 2011 [cited January 3, 2013]. Available at: www.aAHSC.org/download/77168/data/professionalism.pdf

7. Flexner A. *Medical Education in the United States and Canada: a report to the Carnegie Foundation for the Advancement of Teaching* [Bulletin Number Four]. New York, NY; 1910 [cited January 3, 2013]. Available at: www.carnegiefoundation.org/sites/default/files/elibrary/Carnegie_Flexner_Report.pdf

8. Royal College of Physicians (RCP). *Doctors in Society: medical professionalism in a changing world. Report of a Working Party of the Royal College of Physicians of London*. London: RCP; 2005.

9. The Joint Commission. Behaviors that undermine a culture of safety. *Sentinel Event Alert*. 2008; 40.

10. *Center for Professionalism and Peer Support*. Boston, MA: Brigham and Women's Hospital. 2012. Available at: www.brighamandwomens.org/medical_professionals/career/cpps/ (accessed January 3, 2013).

11. Suchman AL. Organizations as machines, organizations as conversations: two core metaphors and their consequences. *Med Care*. 2011; **49**(Suppl.): S4–8.

12. Federation of State Medical Boards of the United States. *Report of the Special Committee on Professional Conduct and Ethics*. Dallas, TX: Federation of State Medical Boards of the United States: 2000.

13. Rosenstein AH, O'Daniel M. A survey of the impact of disruptive behaviors and communication defects on patient safety. *Jt Comm J Qual Patient Saf*. 2008; **34**(8): 464–71.

14. Smetzer JL, Cohen MR. Intimidation: practitioners speak up about this unresolved problem. *Jt Comm J Qual Patient Saf*. 2005; **31**(10): 594–9.

15. Rosenstein AH, O'Daniel M. Impact and implications of disruptive behavior in the perioperative arena. *J Am Coll Surg*. 2006; **203**(1): 96–105.

16. Whittemore A; New England Society for Vascular Surgery. The impact of professionalism on safe surgical care. *J Vasc Surg*. 2007; **45**(2): 415–19.

17. Felblinger DM. Incivility and bullying in the workplace and nurses' shame responses. *J Obstet Gynecol Neonatal Nurs*. 2008; **37**(2): 234–42.

18. Heifitz RA, Linsky M. When leadership spells danger: leading meaningful change in education takes courage, commitment, and political savvy. *Educ Leadership*. 2004; **61**(7): 33–7.

19. Waterman AD, Garbutt J, Hazel E, *et al*. The emotional impact of medical errors on practicing physicians in the United States and Canada. *Jt Comm J Qual Patient Saf*. 2007; **33**(8): 467–76.

20. Hu YY, Fix ML, Hevelone ND, *et al*. Physicians' needs in coping with emotional stressors: the case for peer support. *Arch Surg*. 2011; **147**(3): 212–17.

21. Gallagher TH, Studdert D, Levinson W. Disclosing harmful medical errors to patients. *N Engl J Med*. 2007; **356**(26): 2713–19.

22. Mello MM, Gallagher TH. Malpractice reform: opportunities for leadership by health care institutions and liability insurers. *N Engl J Med*. 2010; **362**(15): 1353–6.

23. Mastroianni AC, Mello MM, Sommer S, *et al*. The flaws in state 'apology' and 'disclosure'

laws dilute their intended impact on malpractice suits. *Health Aff (Millwood)*. 2010; **29**(9): 1611–19.

24. *Courage and Renewal Programs*. Seattle, WA: Center for Courage and Renewal; 2012. Available at: www.couragerenewal.org/programs (accessed January 3, 2013).

25. Emanuel EJ, Pearson S. Physician autonomy and health care reform. *JAMA*. 2012; **307**(4): 367–8.

Cultivating Compassion

COMPASSION IS A FUNDAMENTAL CHARACTERISTIC OF A WISE PERSON. Compassion is one characteristic that differentiates intelligence from wisdom. One might expect that compassion comes naturally to health-care providers and health-care organizations. In some measure, it does. But in reality, being compassionate, particularly in times of stress, constraints, competing values, or moral conflict, is difficult. Like reflection, compassion is more of a practice, a discipline, than a decision. Compassion comes from deep inside ourselves and our communities, practice must be fostered and nurtured daily if we are to be able to mobilize and manifest it in all circumstances toward all people.

In the story that follows, Beth Lown describes one very powerful approach to fostering compassion in our health-care organizations. Schwartz Center Rounds grew out of one patient's experience of compassion. Kenneth Schwartz was a lawyer, husband, father, and cancer patient who recognized the critical role that compassion played in his own illness experience. He created a foundation that seeks to cultivate and foster compassion in caregivers and now supports "Schwartz Center Rounds" in hospitals across the country.

In her chapter on fostering compassion, Dorrie Fontaine describes an intentional process of fostering compassionate care in a large academic health system. One partner in this school of nursing is Monica Sharma, who brought her years of experience with the United Nations to the project. In 20 years of dealing with highly charged situations to improve the lives of millions of vulnerable women and children, Sharma developed an approach to creating change that helped apply the deepest wisdom of leaders and their compassion to seemingly irresolvable conflicts, and helped find solutions to seemingly unsolvable problems. Sharma, Fontaine, and colleagues applied this model to bring together formal and informal leaders throughout a large health system to empower them in fostering compassion in their areas of influence.

A Story: Holding One Another

Beth A. Lown

I had been working at Mount Auburn Hospital, a regional teaching hospital of Harvard Medical School, for many years when I first learned about the Schwartz Center for Compassionate Healthcare from an elderly couple who nominated me for the Center's annual compassionate caregiver award. I took care of both the wife and her husband who had a protracted, complicated illness and who ultimately died at home. I was certain that he had survived as long as he had only because of the tenacity and devotion of his wife. I made frequent home visits to the couple during his long dying process to sit and listen, to support his wife, tweak his regimen, and make decisions together. But I knew too that I was learning profound lessons from them about the meaning of enduring love and I was drawn toward their warmth.

When the chief executive officer of Mount Auburn Hospital, Jeanette Clough (a nurse by training), asked me to consider initiating Schwartz Center Rounds at the hospital, I had a good sense of the integrity of the program's origins. The Schwartz Center Rounds program, launched in 1997 at one site, now takes place in over 300 sites in the United States and England, providing a multidisciplinary and interprofessional, highly interactive forum to discuss the challenging emotional and social issues that arise during patient care and the impact these issues have on patients, families, and clinical caregivers. With the guidance of the Schwartz Center, we engaged a social worker to be our Rounds facilitator and created a Rounds planning committee that included the directors of medical and surgical education, the hospital chaplain, representatives from nursing, social work, house staff, and other interested clinicians. Our goals were to provide a safe forum for discussion, to provide and receive support, to build communication across professions and disciplines, to facilitate the expression and understanding of multiple perspectives, to model for learners behaviors of nonjudgmental listening and respect, and to return with renewed compassion and insight to the patients we serve. We began the Schwartz Center Rounds program in 2005 and our sessions have been consistently well attended. Now that the program is well established in

---

our hospital, people come to me often with stories of patients and families, both challenging and joyful, that they would like to discuss in community.

A recent, particularly challenging Schwartz Center Rounds session focused on the death of a young child who had been found unresponsive and was brought to the emergency room by ambulance. Members of the emergency room staff and the hospital chaplain each shared their experiences of that day. In an unsteady voice, the emergency room physician, a young mother herself, described her pain at having to stop the resuscitation effort after it became clear the child was not responding.

The child's mother arrived shortly thereafter and her piercing wails could be heard throughout the emergency department, chilling the souls of all who could hear them. The nurse manager said that as the mother's cries continued, the father arrived. A war veteran, he cursed God for taking his child away after fighting for his country to keep his family safe. The hospital chaplain arrived and held them, humbled in the presence of such grief. The staff found it difficult to manage their grief that day. Those who were able to move on apologized for the delay to the patients who were waiting, but these patients told the staff to take care of this family first. They would wait. The discussion in the Schwartz Center Rounds brought up how clinical caregivers cope with grief, with fear for our own families when confronted by something as incomprehensible as the death of a child, the price of repression of powerful emotions, and the risk of burnout—depersonalization and emotional exhaustion. In the end, we invariably discover strength in sharing these experiences and what has helped us cope individually and collectively.

The Schwartz Center Rounds offer the possibility of understanding the perspectives and experiences of others—a space to deepen empathy for patients, families, and coworkers alike; a safe space for reflection in community. They build a sense of connection and teamwork, diminish hierarchy, and sustain those who attend. I personally feel reconnected with the purpose of medicine and my place in the world after these sessions—to foster compassion, healing relationships, and the health and well-being of our patients, their families, and our communities of care. I know these feelings are shared by others.

5

Cultivating Compassion and Empathy

Dorrie K. Fontaine, Cynda H. Rushton, and Monica Sharma

Introduction

Current challenges in health care require new paradigms of leadership. Some say we have lost the soul of health care. Nurses, physicians, and other health-care providers question their career choices, feeling that the heart that called them to their tasks has been broken. Others point to the business aspects of health care and see how they erode true caring and compassion for our patients, families, communities, and even students. Whether it is the need for creative optimism, a hope for increased self-awareness in ourselves and colleagues, or a plan to harness the talents of the entire health-care workforce, individuals and organizations are craving a new path to leadership and action to relieve human anxiety and suffering. In this chapter we will tell the story of the Compassionate Care and Empathic Leadership Initiative at the University of Virginia (UVA). This initiative was a multidisciplinary effort to infuse compassion into all that we do in the UVA Health System and to inspire and empower compassionate and empathic leadership. The initiative used a model for change, the *Conscious Full-Spectrum Response Model*, which we describe in this chapter, as a way of inspiring an expanded, empowered sense of what it means to be a compassionate and empathic leader. The model suggests that tapping into wisdom and power, shifting systems, and solving problems is one emerging paradigm for leaders in academic health science centers to adopt.

Pamela Ross, physician in the emergency department (ED), shared this perspective on the initiative:

Look up, take courage. Angels are nearer than you think.

—Unknown

Life in the Emergency Department . . . What can I say? It is the location where all forces—good and evil—operate in their maximal capacity. They come to us—by air, by ambulance, by car and old beat-up pickup trucks, by motorcycle and scooter, by foot—through pain, fear, disappointment, trauma, drama, great expectation, anger, illness, illusions, delusions, death and more . . .

To operate compassionately, to minister from the heart, to see the person first—before the disease . . . To take the time to humbly acknowledge the human life that has entered your presence that day . . . To be fully accepting of whatever comes . . . Sometimes it's all enough to knock you over and render you motionless from your own sense of frustration and helplessness . . . To make you pause, hesitate, and wonder if you have what you need to give to that person in that moment. And to worry if, in any given moment, you will be swallowed whole by the process or the simply overwhelming condition of the masses.

Then you look up. You look up and you catch a glimpse of him walking in the direction of the next patient he must see. Your colleague, Jonathan, that stellar nurse who carries fierce compassion as his personal motto . . . Jonathan who is dedicated, committed, and working in full collaboration with you and others in a powerful network known as the Compassionate Care and Empathic Leadership Initiative. And in the time it takes to look up—the peace you thought had left you declares itself. You breathe in, you breathe out and suddenly—it's like a brand new day has just begun, with brand new mercy. "Look up, take courage. Angels are nearer than you think." That is the strength of the initiative for me.

Why Foster Compassion and Empathy?

If we truly practiced with compassion and empathy, what would the health-care system look like? How would we be transformed? How might this change the outcomes for patients and families and the students we teach?

Compassion

Compassion in health care is an attribute that can be expressed in personal action and even by an institution. A nurse or physician is said to be compassionate or to practice with compassion. An institution may have a reputation for delivering its services and programs in a compassionate manner or upholding compassion as a core value and may express this attribute through the combined actions of its personnel or in its policies. To be compassionate is an essential aspect of wise persons. The absence of this attribute may also too often be visible—we take note of people and organizations that lack compassion. But what is compassion, and how do we foster it?

Compassion has both affective and motivational dimensions.[1] Salzberg[2] notes that compassion taken literally from the Pali and Sanskrit word *karma* means "experiencing a trembling or quivering of the heart in response to a being's pain." This feeling deep inside arises as empathy toward the situation of the other and motivates a person to action that reflects the virtue of compassion. This is the visible dimension of compassion.

Compassion without action is meaningless. It is not enough to respond to the suffering of the other by engaging empathy; action aimed at relieving suffering is needed. Without the motivation to act, compassion is reduced to an affective experience alone. Bonhoeffer's notion of "cheap grace"[3] may suggest an analogous concept of "cheap compassion." Cheap grace means that individuals might attend religious services, for example, and still not pay attention to how they treat others. "Cheap compassion" then could be when individuals claim to be compassionate, and yet their lack of action or inattentiveness suggests otherwise. "Costly compassion," like "costly grace," indicates that the person is changed by the compassionate acts; it costs the person something to respond to the human condition of suffering. We do not wish leaders to use "cheap compassion." To be compassionate requires awareness and being fully aware occurs when hearts are open. Anxiety and suffering are all around us and call for a response that is grounded in creating the conditions for compassion to arise.[1]

Compassion can be fostered by watching skillful health-care providers who understand their own ways of coming to compassion and share this knowledge with others. There is a need to know how to watch and what to look for. According to Back and colleagues,[4] contemplative traditions suggest that compassion is transmitted through a quality of mind and requires active intentional mental processes.

Consider this compassionate awareness of a third-year nursing student:

I followed the chaplain. When I met up with him he had just served a family who lost their second son within months. He said that he wanted to go cry somewhere, but we continued seeing patients. We swooped through the emergency room, but it was uneventful at that time. Then we went through the ICUs [intensive care units] and visited patients who he had a relationship with. He was paged to a room with a man who was being emergently intubated. The look of fear on this man's face was unforgettable. He was drowning and was alone. A team rushed around him, but nobody was talking to him. The chaplain was booted to the hallway. I know that they needed the space, but it seemed that there were extraneous people in the room. I thought that the chaplain could have better used their space. I will keep that in mind if I ever have a patient who desires the chaplain's presence and prioritize the chaplain's spot in the room if possible.

In this story, the student, who is quite early in her education, is already exhibiting an awareness of situation, context, activating empathy, and compassion. She considers the place of the patient who is "drowning," in her words, but also the chaplain. If nursing and medical students can truly notice patients and health-care providers with this level of attention, there is hope for the broken health-care system. In many situations, we can pause to consider thoughtfully our response before reacting.[5] We can choose kindness, listening, and action or we may be abrupt, cut others off with interruptions, or fail to act because of fear. If vast numbers of health-care workers in an institution do not work from a place of stillness, insight, and inquiry, then an entire organization may suffer as their patients surely will, from poor-quality care. The institution may earn a bad reputation. Compassion is not a choice but a necessary ingredient in caring for patients and families. Organizations need to choose compassion. Halifax[1] notes that compassion is not a luxury; it is a necessity for our well-being, resilience, and even our very survival.

Leaders need to *be* compassionate and *act* with compassion. Why? Leadership experts, especially in the business arena, often encourage firm and decisive action and, above all, managing the bottom line. While health care seems different, these traits are also needed, and are not necessarily incompatible. This may seem counterintuitive at first. However, stories and data suggest that all these traits in various forms are needed to provide a high-quality, safe environment where patients and families continue to choose their care and providers. The challenge is to cultivate these capacities and create wise leaders as essential to health-care cultures.

Consider these examples of lack of compassion and how it may hurt the bottom line. A nurse manager in a busy academic health science center might have a reputation for playing favorites, not listening to newer staff or paying attention to medical residents, spending much time in meetings and being largely "invisible" otherwise. The adverse impact of these behaviors may include high turnover of nurses, lack of standards for quality care, patient and family complaints, and even mistreatment of students and poor patient outcomes. This surely will affect the hospital's financial status if patients choose to receive their care elsewhere. A surgeon may display a lack of compassion in the operating room by routinely shouting at others and carry this behavior into the intensive care unit. If a lack of compassion can create this cascade of abuse and sadness, then compassionate leadership needs to be a restorative goal. Choosing first-line leaders and managers for their ability to manifest compassionate action would seem to be essential and aligned with business goals as well. Selecting employees based on their ability to be compassionate during times of joy and pain then requires us to infuse skills in cultivating compassion in interprofessional health sciences students, hire for compassion, and find ways to recognize a lack of compassion and incentivize wiser behaviors.

While the capacity for awareness of self and other may be innately human (*Homo sapiens*), the full development of capacity is not automatic. For most people, the capacity to be deeply aware of their own experience or another's experience must be cultivated through practices and processes that teach us how to be still inside—how to quiet our minds, sense our bodies, and tap into an innate, deep well of wisdom and creativity that can serve us and others in extraordinary ways. With these practices and processes, we learn to be thoughtful, watchful, and observant. We discover the causes of our suffering, and new possibilities for eliminating those causes. The more we change ourselves, the more we can serve others and change the systems that deplete us.

Empathy

Empathy is a necessary precondition for compassion. Practicing with empathy means putting yourself in the shoes of another. It is a fundamental people skill and a central component of emotional intelligence.[6] Drayton[7] sees empathy as an essential component of leading change and generating results. He founded the world renowned Ashoka Foundation for social entrepreneurs worldwide, and the membership includes Mohammad Yunus, a Nobel Prize winner. The foundation's program "Activating Empathy" has led to scores of innovations for communities and institutions.[7] Not judging, staying open, and deep listening are keys to empathy. Nurses and physicians need to be attuned to patients, of course, but also to each other and all members of the team. Because some do this better than others, empathy should be role-modeled, taught, and fostered by empathic leaders. One of the UVA deans invited consultants to work with a particular hospital department after a series of communication "mishaps" that could suggest a lack of empathy. I inquired why the talk was titled *Advanced Listening*, and the dean noted that if advertised as just *Listening*, no one would attend, because these colleagues all believe they are advanced. The room was packed that evening and it was a successful event that included role-playing and honest sharing. The dean was right.

An example of being attuned and cultivating empathy toward fellow providers is exhibited in this story from our UVA ED. One nurse, Jonathan Bartels, noticed that typically after a patient's death in the busy ED, staff usually felt demoralized, guilty, and sad and then quickly left one another to go on to the next patient. Instituting the "pause" became a compassionate intervention due to this nurse's empathy for his colleagues. Here is his story:

> I noted that when people die after a traumatic incident, a code, often I would see surgeons and docs and nurses walk away in frustration, throw their gloves off in a defeatist attitude, not recognizing that the patient was a human being we worked on saving. So after these deaths I decided it would be a good thing to stop, pause and do a moment of silence. Just stopping; honoring the patient in your own way,

> in silence. Dr. Y from the trauma service loves it. We have even had family members participate.

Note where the intervention of the "pause" came from—one nurse's empathy and compassion for colleagues and the ability to restore meaning to an event that could become routine in the ED and harden feelings, leading to exhaustion and burnout. The benefit of this practice has spread throughout the hospital, with one nurse telling the story of an anesthesiologist on one of the medical floors, who after a patient died, suggested "could we just pause for a minute like they do in the ED?" This story is being told across the hospital. It reminds us of how we need positive stories that encourage the heart and need to be told. As Lopez[8] wrote in his book *Crow and Weasel*:

> Remember only this one thing. The stories people tell have a way of taking care of them. If stories come to you, care for them. And learn to give them away where they are needed. Sometimes a person needs a story more than food to stay alive. That is why we put these stories in each other's memories. This is how people take care of themselves.

Compassion is a demanding practice. It combines the strength of a stable mind and emotions (a "strong back") with an open heart ("soft front").[9] What is required is the cultivation of these conditions within oneself to be stable, clear and non-reactive in the midst of challenging circumstances. A strong back is needed to withstand the pressures that can exist in health-care systems that are not designed to be patient or clinician friendly. The same quality is needed when the suffering of our patients overwhelms us. A soft front is supported by a connection to the meaning of our work, our intentions with openheartedness and a generous spirit. It is the balance of these states that allow compassionate action to arise. These qualities are cultivated through principled action and sustained practices aimed at stabilizing the mental and emotional continuum, focusing attention, and inviting insight.[1,5] Compassion is not only an ideal, it is a *way of being* in our professional world that embodies these values and intentions.

Application to Leadership and to Health-Care System Change at the University of Virginia

At the UVA Medical Center, we are cultivating the mindsets, intentions, and qualities of clinicians who can *authentically* do this work through the application of a model of leadership used throughout the world to turn breakdowns into breakthroughs, and by tapping into our deepest wisdom, to shift systems and solve problems.[10,11]

We Get Started: Attending the Upaya Institute 2009

In order to be able to shift systems, there needs to be grounding in a shared mindset and orientation to the unfolding process. In 2009 an initial interprofessional group of 10 health-care providers from UVA attended the 8-day program offered by the Upaya Institute, called Being with Dying (www.upaya.org/bwd/). The Upaya program focused on the cultivation of the necessary mental qualities and practical skills that allow caregivers to effectively accompany dying people and their families through the experience of a catastrophic illness and/or the dying process using self-awareness, mentoring, and sustained practice skills.[5] Now, a total of 45 interdisciplinary UVA colleagues have attended the 1-week Upaya program over a 4-year period, building a foundation and capacity for our Compassionate Care and Empathic Leadership Initiative. After a year of discussions in 2009 with a colleague, Cynda Rushton, we decided to focus our efforts on enhancing the work environment and creating resilient practitioners and students. During this time we also supported a compassionate lecture series bringing further explorations and awareness to our community. Jon Kabat-Zinn, Roshi Joan Halifax, and Sharon Salzberg were invited to UVA to share their expertise.

Following an assessment of the goals of key stakeholders within the University and Health System, a consensus emerged to integrate current programs and initiatives into a larger effort we entitled the "Compassionate Care and Empathic Leadership Initiative." Recognizing the need to ground this work in the stability of mindful and compassionate action, key stakeholders from nursing, medicine, social work, chaplains, educators, practitioners of integrative therapies and mindfulness, and the broader community were engaged. In 2010, we invited Monica Sharma to join with Cynda Rushton to help design, frame, and implement the emerging initiative. Monica Sharma is an internationally renowned physician and former 20-year director of Leadership and Capacity Development

TABLE 5.1 Vision and Mission of the Compassionate Care Initiative, University of Virginia

"Reducing human suffering by cultivating compassionate people and systems"

Vision: To reduce human suffering and promote health and well-being through the creation of innovative, scalable, adaptable models of health care that incorporate practices that invite stillness, inquiry, and insight and are grounded in compassionate action and empathic leadership.

Mission: To develop clinical, educational, and research initiatives, focusing first on systems to optimize quality of life for patients and their families, that incorporate compassionate action and empathic leadership into personal behavior, interprofessional interactions and encounters with patients and families across the lifespan.

We have worked with a compassionate care frame of problem solving, pattern creating, and power and passion to design a program for transformation and results. This model asks each of us to think differently and to act with integrity. In the process we are creating new pattern shifts:

- from scarcity to abundance
- from fragmentation to wholeness and integration
- from isolation to inclusion and connectedness
- from fear to courage.

At our series of workshops the goals are to:

- envision and outline actions for accomplishing a different future for care, in the context of life-threatening illness and end-of-life care in health institutions and communities
- deepen our understanding of ourselves and sharpen our strategies to create space for synergy
- distinguish methods and practices that allow people to shift perceptions for new actions to be taken
- know the power of commitment, personal responsibility as a freedom to act, and the power of taking a stand
- engage in a process to better distinguish immediate, systemic, and root causes of inadequate care and envisage approaches that address the three domains simultaneously
- view ourselves as pattern makers, not only problem solvers—as leaders of the future
- identify breakthrough initiatives to engage people and organizations for social change, in constructing a new social reality and inspiring action.

at the United Nations. Her work has transformed some of the world's most challenging problems into solutions. She developed a new paradigm to address large-scale problems such as HIV/AIDS in Africa, land mines in the Middle East, and other global issues. It represents a unique response model, first described in the 2007 paper "Personal to Planetary Transformation," and more recently in a paper on transformational leaders.[11] The model is a way to create sustainable change by seeing the world differently, identifying new patterns, and asking all to identify and acknowledge their unique strength and power. Cynda Rushton is a Professor of Nursing, Pediatrics, and Bioethics at the Johns Hopkins University, and has extensive experience in large-scale projects that bring patients, families, and interprofessionals together to address aspects of health care. Together they inspired UVA clinicians, faculty, and our community to engage in an ongoing process to create and sustain change and solve problems. The initial challenge we chose to address was improving care of those with serious illness and those dying in the Charlottesville community. Table 5.1 provides a description of the vision and mission of the Compassionate Care and Empathic Leadership Initiative.

The Conscious Full-Spectrum Model: A Description

The model that framed the efforts of Sharma and Rushton is described as a "response" model. The name implies that we can consciously respond to a challenge by using three frames that create knowledge, understanding, and wisdom. There are many frameworks that enhance understanding, but we know that understanding phenomena, or the set of factors that give rise to a problem, is necessary but not sufficient to generate results or transformational change. The model encourages us to stop reacting automatically and without full knowledge, and to respond from our deepest wisdom. An important feature of this model is aligning the various components that are needed for a response. Too often these dimensions of leadership and elements of a problem are fragmented, and this combination does not produce optimal solutions. Wisdom leadership, however, can be cultivated to create systemic shifts and solve problems. Perhaps Jerry White,[12] the current US Deputy Assistant Secretary for Conflict Stabilization Operations, identifies the components of the model in the clearest manner. White[12] described how Sharma's model assisted him to align leaders to work on the elimination of land mines in Israel, Jordan, and Palestine after he lost a leg to

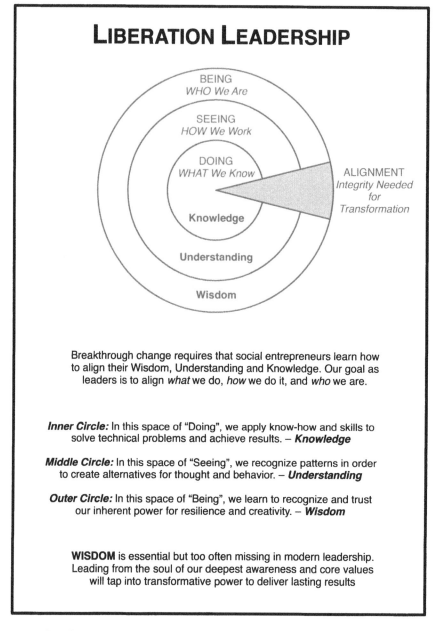

FIGURE 5.1 The Conscious Full-Spectrum Response Model: liberation leadership[12]

one in 1984. He noted that many gifted individuals are misaligned in how they approach work and life and he personally had many failures in this effort before he adopted the model. White met Sharma and was introduced to this model at a workshop at the University of Notre Dame Mendoza College of Business in 2009. He stated that it was not until he focused on the model that he was able to "tap into the power of wisdom" and act generously to bring disparate groups together who had shared values. White identifies the model, stating that "Doing-seeing-being" leads to knowledge, understanding, and wisdom.

The inner circle depicted in Figure 5.1 is the space of "Doing," where we apply know-how and skills to solve technical problems and achieve results or knowledge. The middle circle space he refers to as "Seeing," where we recognize patterns in order to create alternatives for thought and behavior, which is understanding. Finally, the outer circle is the space of "Being," where we learn to recognize and trust our inherent power for resilience and creativity, which is wisdom.

Too often frameworks imply that working on oneself to gain inner strength and competencies through various self-help programs is the only key to success. Other change models focus on how to fix broken systems, become "change warriors," [vigorous champions for needed change] to benefit the organization. Still others from business suggest a methodical approach of clear goal direction. These are partial responses alone and do not account for barriers that shift or results that sustain. The model is called a full-spectrum response for this reason. The strength of the Conscious Full-Spectrum Response model is that it identifies the faulty logic of each framework used alone where success is fleeting or uncommon. For example, if a person has learned about contemplative practices and decides to use meditation and mindfulness techniques to become more focused, this is a strength. However, unless they consciously use these skills to shift systems that create the barriers to results and outcomes, it is just a changed feeling or attitude for that one person. The full potential for a societal problem or concern is not realized.

The Conscious Full-Spectrum Response model for leadership, by contrast, is intended to explicate how all of the vital elements need to be invoked synchronously and synergistically to respond to a particular challenging situation. It combines identifying results or solving problems (inner circle) with use of inner wisdom and power (outer circle) to shift systems (middle circle to sustain change). It trains for a deeply reflective way of thinking and sourcing wisdom that informs action by removing the multiple barriers to solutions that work. Alignment of all three circles is essential. Figure 5.2 adapts the model for creating resilience in the workplace and supports the Compassionate Care and Empathic Leadership initiative. It is this full-spectrum response to challenges that has been especially useful in approaching challenges engaged at UVA.

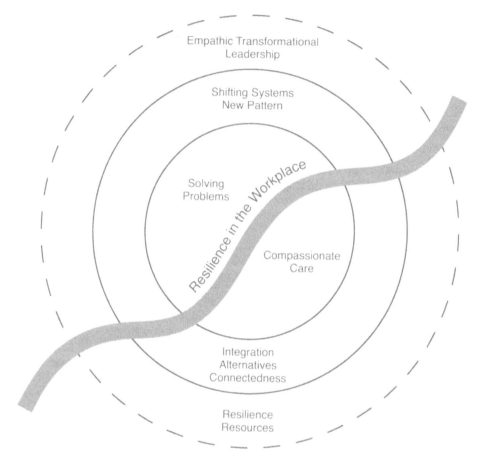

FIGURE 5.2 A framework for resilience in the workplace: compassionate care and empathic leadership[13]

A good example from this initiative involves Jonathan Bartels, who appeared in the story told earlier. Jonathan was already a compassionate nurse with a deep practice of contemplation, giving exquisite care to patients and families every day. But it was not until he joined our initiative and found others who shared his values, including physician, chaplain and social worker colleagues in the ED, that "the pause" was born. This intervention came from seeing a problem with fresh eyes and having the courage to start a new tradition. The model effectively fosters the deepest wisdom, which is our common source of humanity around which we all connect. We are using the model to provide improved quality of life for those with serious illness and those at the end of life. Monica Sharma's results-oriented approach of solving problems through sourcing inner wisdom and power to shift systems is creating a new army of confident leaders.

Each Compassionate Care and Empathetic Leadership Initiative workshop has been designed by Sharma and Rushton to facilitate progress on goals identified by the leaders at UVA. The workshop format always starts off with a contemplative mindfulness moment and an exercise of "Who Am I—What Do I Stand For—What is My Unique Contribution?" to enable each participant to stand in their own power and commit to action. Sharma's enlightened stories about heroes from her work around the world[11] who have the qualities, advanced abilities, described as "un-messable-with-ness" and "bozo-ability" (acting in spite of fear) have captured the hearts of these leaders who vow to meet problems head on, and change systems by removing barriers, all by sourcing their deepest wisdom. Topics covered include how to deeply listen, how to engage and enroll others in a shared commitment, and how to turn inevitable breakdowns into breakthroughs. Throughout the intercession work between meetings, we are asked to notice how we may show up differently to our colleagues and our work. One oncology-nursing professor noticed this and reported:

> Shifts in myself? An ability to pull myself back when losing compassion and nurture relationships. I try to be supportive, encouraging and nurturing to everyone I interact with. What energizes me is to remember strategies I have learned in the workshops here to keep compassionate care a priority.

Transformations occur and are shared. When the pediatric palliative care group recognized that children did not have the same access to services that adults received, the group actually raised money, and lobbied to hire a pediatric nurse practitioner to work with physician colleagues on this issue. This idea had been discussed for over 5 years without any action. Our initiative made action possible. We transformed a breakdown into a breakthrough and now children with life-limiting illness are better served. Here is what a community pediatrician shared:

> Being a part of the initiative helps me lead from strengths and core values. I've learned to identify strengths in myself and recognize them in others. Gives me an opportunity to think about who I am and who I can be as a leader. Helps me to see the effects of engaging people's commitments to a project and their core values. Creates synergy in a group. We have been able to extend the palliative care with

> children and improve the services in the hospital and the community through partnerships. What keeps me coming back (to the meetings) is sharing the energy and having a place to think about and explore your own passion for what you do but also sustain and draw up the passion in other people.

In between the workshops or intersessions, integration of practices in compassionate action councils was supported with monthly meetings. After 2 years of workshops held every few months, the Compassionate Care and Empathetic Leadership Initiative has demonstration projects and action councils in seven areas: (1) palliative care, (2) cancer, (3) the emergency department, (4) education, (5) pediatrics, (6) the transitional care hospital, and (7) a lactation group. Nurses, physicians, community members, social workers, chaplains, and educators populate these action councils. As one member stated:

> I am able to lead from a more grounded place. I have the ability to be more open and willing to make change. I have grown by getting a good sense of who I am, "stand in your power," be fearless and limitless ... no matter what obstacles, if we can just get people on board with us, there are no limits to what we can do. "No" means "not yet."

We are committed to becoming and creating empathic leaders who guide others with compassion. Table 5.2 lists Sharma's literacies of an empathic leader.

TABLE 5.2 Literacies of an Empathic Leader

Self-Awareness

Emotional self-awareness
Reading one's own emotions and recognizing their impact, using "gut sense" to guide decisions
Accurate self-assessment
Knowing one's strengths and limits
Self-confidence
A sound sense of one's self-worth and capabilities

Fostering Leadership

Seeking out potential leaders and creating opportunities for their development

Being a leader while actively supporting the leadership of others

Embracing one's social, professional, and personal profiles and moving flexibly among them as required

Champion the human dignity of all

Building Partnerships and Networks for Change

Cultivating and maintaining a web of effective, empathetic, and ethical relationships, networks, and constellations

Actively fostering partnerships that generate principled action and results; providing the necessary support, coordination, collaboration; maximizing synergy in partnerships

Speaking Out and Speaking Up

Based on self-understanding, empathy, and ethics, having the courage to speak up for actions that result in long-term business success, as well as global sustainability

Creating a supporting environment where others can also speak up, take risks, and make mistakes

Creating Sustainable Systems Alternatives

Recognizing the invisible, multiple patterns and systems that shape societal and global situations and actions; recognizing interdependence

Distinguishing, designing, and delivering on actions simultaneously in real time that (1) source from self-understanding, empathy, and ethics; (2) manifest sustainable change and shift systems; and (3) solve problems

Unleashing the power of effective creativity, being a pattern maker while simultaneously sourcing wisdom

Creating Platforms for Transformation

Create transformational spaces within routine action

Shift processes and the way business is done or transacted

Conflict Transformation

Sourcing self-awareness, empathy, and ethics to resolve conflicts and create new relationship patterns

One of the skills learned in the workshops was how to transform a breakdown into a breakthrough. Clinicians found this very powerful tool and have practiced this throughout the academic health system. From a neonatal intensive care nurse:

> Breakdowns are a demonstration of compassion and commitment to change. We had an infant dying and needed to switch to more comfort care rather than pushing forward with medical interventions. Over the weekend the nurses, nurse practitioners and physicians and the unit secretary were not sure how to handle the case now that the baby was not going to survive. We had to break the rules and let more visitors in for the family's sake. Let them eat food in the room. Some did not understand this and had problems with rules being broken. We needed an individualized care plan. Bottom line was giving a family memories that they can think of with warmth and appreciation. I did not walk away.

The positive response to the Sharma and Rushton workshops has created increased capacity for leadership in fostering compassion and empathy. It also serves to build community in truly integrated new ways. Hear this message from a palliative care physician:

> One of the problems when you work in a big institution is people work in silos and do not have a sense of shared vision. People can get lonely and burnt out. Having a sense of shared community makes everyone feel more energized and inspired. . . . this initiative helps to take things that seem like intractable problems and reframe them. Instead of being debilitated or hopeless, it gave a sense of energy.

The workshops have moved us along a journey that we liken to the serpentine wall that Thomas Jefferson designed for the gardens and the lawn at the University he created 200 years ago. These walls are one brick thick and curve or snake around the gardens. Their strength and beauty lies in the one-brick thickness. Serpentine walls are stronger than normal straight walls, because they buttress themselves. The Compassionate Care and Empathic Leadership Initiative has used this imagery to capture the power of each of us when joined together. We are committed to taking our learnings to scale.

The pause in the ED as well as the ED's weekly mindfulness and medical review programs have yielded real outcomes.[14] We are collecting stories of how we have changed the landscape and ourselves by asking these questions: How have you grown during this process? What shifts have you noticed in yourself? What shifts have you noticed in your colleagues and your environment? What energizes you and keeps you going? What projects have you implemented? How has your project contributed to a healthy work environment, policies and structures, and community? Results can be seen on a video titled *Compassionate Care*.[15]

Summary

This chapter has explored the qualities of compassion and empathy and their joint relevance to leadership. Leaders face enormous challenges as they personally embody and attempt to suffuse compassion and empathy throughout the systems they lead. One way that leaders can connect to their compassionate selves is through the use of the Conscious Full-Spectrum Response Model. We have used this model to foster the wise traits of compassion and empathy and their connection in leaders. Connections made, we have inspired leaders through the Compassionate Care and Empathic Leadership Initiative to improve the care of those with serious illness at the end-of-life by fostering compassion and empathy in themselves and others, creating resilient leaders and a strengthened self-buttressing health-care system.

References

1. Halifax J. The precious necessity of compassion. *J Pain Symptom Manage*. 2011; **41**(1): 146–53.
2. Salzberg S. *Lovingkindness: the revolutionary art of happiness*. Boston, MA: Shambala Publications; 1995.
3. Metaxas E. *Bonhoeffer: pastor, martyr, prophet, spy*. Nashville, TN: Thomas Nelson; 2010.
4. Back AL, Bauer-Wu SM, Rushton CH, *et al*. Compassionate silence in the patient-clinician encounter: a contemplative approach. *J Palliat Med*. 2009; **12**(12): 1113–17.
5. Rushton CH. Ethical discernment and action: the art of pause. *AACN Adv Crit Care*. 2009; **20**(1): 108–11.
6. Goleman D. *Emotional Intelligence*. New York, NY: Bantam Books; 1995.
7. Drayton B. *Everyone a Changemaker*. Arlington, VA: Ashoka; 2012. Available at: www.ashoka.org/files/innovations8.5x11FINAL_0.pdf January 2, 2013.
8. Lopez B. *Crow and Weasel*. New York, NY: North Point; 1989.
9. Halifax J. *Being with Dying: cultivating compassion and fearlessness in the presence of death*. Boston, MA: Shambala Publications; 2008.
10. Sharma M. Personal to planetary transformation. *Kosmos*. 2007; Fall/Winter: 31–5.

11. Sharma M. Contemporary leaders of courage and compassion: competencies and inner capacities. Transformational leaders series—part one. *Kosmos*. 2012; Spring/Summer: 4–11.

12. White J. Explosive leadership: what landmines teach us about liberation and leadership. Transformational leaders series—part two. *Kosmos*. 2012; Spring/Summer: 12–20.

13. Fontaine D.K. Standing in my power: Becoming a fearless dean. *Kosmos*. 2012; Fall/Winter: 39–42.

14. Cunningham T, Bartels J, Grant C, *et al*. Mindfulness and medical review: a grassroots approach to improving work/life balance and nursing retention in a level I trauma center emergency department. *J Emerg Nurs*. 2013; **39**(2): 200–2.

15. *UVa School of Nursing's Compassionate Care and Empathetic Leadership Initiative* [video]. Charlottesville: University of Virginia School of Nursing; 2013. Available at: http://vimeo.com/54874862

Connecting and Leading with Others

WISDOM RESEARCHER JOHN MEACHAM NOTES THAT WISDOM DOES NOT begin in our own heads, but rather in interpersonal relationships, learned and maintained in a community. As he states,

> in a wisdom atmosphere, there is a supportive network of interpersonal relations in which doubts, uncertainties and questions can be openly expressed, in which ambiguities and contradictions can be tolerated so that individuals are not forced to adopt the defensive position of too confident knowing.

In addition, wise persons understand the limits of one person's knowing, and thus comprehend the power of teams. In the chapter that follows, Jody Hoffer Gittell and Anthony Suchman describe the importance of relationships in leading the academic health science center, and how fostering relationality can enhance wise decision making and improve outcomes.

6

Connecting and Leading
with Others

Jody Hoffer Gittell and Anthony L. Suchman

LEADERSHIP IS INSTRUMENTAL FOR ACHIEVING ORGANIZATIONAL change, whether through the exercise of power or influence. In this chapter we introduce the concept of relational leadership and suggest it is particularly essential for achieving change in the current health-care context, given the growing evidence that well-functioning work relationships help to drive the quality and efficiency of health-care delivery, and the well-being of care providers and their patients. Academic medicine, in particular, faces the challenge of fragmented care due to strong disciplinary silos and competing commitments. We argue that relational leadership, relational coordination, and relational coproduction are three *mutually supportive* forms of reciprocal interrelating based on shared goals, shared knowledge, and mutual respect, that together drive high performance. We present a case study that illustrates the importance of relational leadership for implementing family-centered rounds at Riley Children's Hospital.

Introduction

Leadership is instrumental for achieving organizational change, whether through the exercise of power or influence. Using influence to achieve organizational change requires articulating a vision that others want to achieve. In this chapter we show that influence is a relational process, and that relational leadership is a process of reciprocal influence between leaders and those they lead. More specifically, relational leadership is a process of reciprocal interrelating between leaders and those they lead, achieved through the development of shared goals, shared knowledge, and mutual respect.[1] Relational leaders create influence in two primary ways: (1) by developing shared goals, shared knowledge, and mutual respect *with* others and (2) by developing shared goals, shared knowledge, and mutual respect *among* others. Relational leaders support the development of relational coordination among workers, as well as relational coproduction between workers and the clients, families, and communities that they serve. Also known as relationship-centered care,[2] these relational processes together drive positive performance outcomes such as high-quality care with fewer wasted resources and greater well-being of those involved.

In health systems around the world, reform efforts are focused on achieving higher quality and greater cost-effectiveness. The motivation for these efforts is the rise of health-care costs due to the aging of the population and the increase in chronic illness. Policy-makers and leaders are beginning to converge on a core set of solutions, most of which call for increased coordination among care providers across professional boundaries.[3] Relational leadership is therefore particularly relevant for achieving change in the current context, given the growing evidence that well-functioning work relationships help to drive both quality and efficiency of health-care delivery, while fostering the well-being of care providers and their patients.

In this chapter we explore these relational processes, then present a case study that illustrates the use of relational leadership to implement family-centered rounds at Riley Hospital for Children in Indianapolis, Indiana. The case study shows how relational leadership led to the sustained implementation of family-centered rounds by fostering relational coordination between physicians, residents, nurses, pharmacists, and social workers, and relational coproduction with the families themselves engaged as partners. We conclude by introducing the Relational Model of Organizational Change and summarizing the role of relational leadership in creating and sustaining positive change.

Relational Leadership

Relational leadership has much in common with related concepts such as distributed leadership, shared leadership, connective leadership, fluid expertise, and leading through humble inquiry. Ancona and Bresman[4] explored the concept of distributed leadership as a form of leadership that is carried out by both formal and informal leaders throughout the organization to facilitate achievement of organizational objectives. They demonstrated that leadership is a form of influence that can be exercised by participants at any level of an organization, and that leaders are most effective when they can inspire others to engage in the responsibilities of leadership rather than attempting to carry out all leadership responsibilities on their own. Distributed leadership thus requires facilitative leadership behaviors more so than directive leadership behaviors, and transformative leaderships behaviors more so than transactional or passive leadership behaviors. Lending support to this perspective, Carson *et al.*[5] found that supportive supervisory behaviors predict greater frontline worker engagement in shared leadership.

Relational leadership as articulated in Gittell and Douglass[6] is characterized by the development of shared goals, shared knowledge, and mutual respect between workers and managers. Relational leadership has much in common with the concept of distributed leadership. However, relational leadership does more than draw upon the expertise and unique perspectives of participants throughout the organization; it also fosters the effective integration of their expertise and perspectives. Participants cocreate and benefit from a more holistic perspective for understanding their own work and making their own decisions. This holistic perspective provides a mechanism through which they manage their interdependence.

Relational leadership also draws on the concept of "connective leadership" as articulated by Lipman-Blumen:[7]

> Connective leadership derives its label from its character of connecting individuals not only to their own tasks and ego drives, but also to those of the group and community that depend upon the accomplishment of mutual goals. It is leadership that connects individuals to others and to others' goals, using a broad spectrum of behavioral strategies. It is leadership that "proceeds from

a premise of connection" and a recognition of networks of relationships that bind society in a web of mutual responsibilities.[8]

Relational leadership is therefore a process of cocreation that requires a particular set of skills, as reflected in Fletcher's[9] concept of "fluid expertise":

> [P]ower and/or expertise shifts from one party to the other, not only over time but in the course of one interaction. This requires two skills. One is a skill in empowering others; an ability to share—in some instances even customizing—one's own reality, skill, knowledge, etc. in ways that made it accessible to others. The other is skill in being empowered: an ability and willingness to step away from the expert role in order to learn from or be influenced by the other.

Willingness to step away from the expert role in order to learn from the other is also known as "leading through humble inquiry."[10] When designated leaders demonstrate this willingness, they help to create a safe space for all participants to set aside egos in order to connect for a shared purpose. Leading through humble inquiry is therefore foundational to the process of relational leadership. Note that leading through humble inquiry does not require one to be humble in the sense of lacking confidence in one's own contributions. To the contrary, leading through humble inquiry requires the confidence to recognize that one's own contributions, however essential, are not sufficient to achieve the desired outcomes given the distribution of relevant expertise and the need for distinct areas of expertise to contribute to a more holistic understanding of the situation.

In Figure 6.1 we see that relational leaders develop relationships *with* others, in such a way that serves to foster relationships *between* others. "Others" can include both colleagues and clients. Relational coordination is simply coordinating work through relationships of shared goals, shared knowledge, and mutual respect with one's colleagues. Relational coproduction is the coproduction of outcomes by workers in partnership with their clients, again through relationships of shared goals, shared knowledge, and mutual respect. Both represent ways of *working together that transform professionalism from the protection of one's exclusive expertise toward a collaborative generative process with potential benefits for all stakeholders.*[11-13]

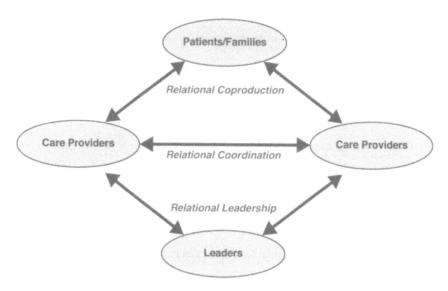

FIGURE 6.1 Relational leadership supporting relational coordination and coproduction

What are Family-Centered Rounds?

Family-centered rounds are a set of processes that call for both relational coordination among care providers, and relational coproduction between those care providers and the families that they serve. Sisterhen et al.[14] define patient- or family-centered rounds as interdisciplinary bedside work rounds in which the patient and family participate as active team members in creating and carrying out the management plan and evaluating the plan's progress and success. These innovative rounds have had some success over the years. Uhlig et al.[15] studied the introduction of a new "interdisciplinary care team" model that included a collaborative communication protocol and daily team rounds at each patient's bedside, and reported a 56% reduction in risk-adjusted mortality for cardiac surgery patients. At Cincinnati Children's Hospital family-centered rounds were initiated on one acute care unit, found to improve communication, shared decision making, offered new learning, and were found to be so successful that it became standard practice on all units.[16] Outcomes of family-centered rounds at Riley Hospital for Children were increased feelings of inclusion and respect and better understanding of their child's care.[17] Based on early evidence, the inclusion of family members in patient-centered rounds was recommended by the American College of Critical Care Medicine's guidelines[18] supporting patient-centered care. However, these published studies provide relatively little insight into the struggles involved in implementing family-centered rounds, or the kinds of leadership required to *achieve and sustain* family-centered rounding as an ongoing organizational practice. The following case study provides these insights.

Family-Centered Rounds at Riley Hospital for Children

In 2008, family-centered rounds were implemented at Riley Hospital for Children under the leadership of Dr. Michele Saysana, a pediatric hospitalist, based on what she and her colleagues had learned from the Cincinnati Children's model. Riley is part of the Indiana University Health system, an 18-hospital system headquartered in Indianapolis with a presence throughout the state. Saysana explained the origin of the idea:

> We used to do bedside rounds but very differently. We would round at the bedside, but it was the old internal medicine model. We talked to each other in front of the patient then told them what we were going to do. Definitely not in ways they would understand. Or we would round in a conference room, then we'd go out and see the patients separately, and try to track down the family. Prior to implementing family-centered rounds on the hospitalist team, one of the other units brought families into the conference room to hear the discussion. They would bring the parents in and tell them what they were going to do that day. But to make families feel more comfortable it's important that we do it on THEIR turf, on THEIR terms. It's less intimidating. We can see the patient too. So now they are doing it this way too.

Residents and medical students are asked to present to the family rather than to the attending physician. Presenting to the family changes the dynamics and the language used, in a way that is beneficial yet highly challenging. According to Saysana:

> We are not allowed to talk the way we do in the conference room. It is SO hard for medical students. It makes them nervous. They are nervous to be presenting to the family anyway, and nervous to be using regular language—they think using medical jargon is a sign of their knowledge. I say no, it tells me even more

if you can translate to the patient. It totally throws them for a loop. Sometimes they even call the patient "the diagnosis." We have to spend time on that. But we let them know that we're like a big safety net. If they get something wrong I will correct it right there but in a way that's respectful. Then the family, the nurse, the social worker, and the pharmacist all understand the plan of care and hear the same plan of care. They know how we explained it so they can continue to reinforce it after the rounds.

The other thing is that everybody is there so everybody hears. That's worth its weight in gold. Especially the families who are having a hard time with social issues—when everybody on the team hears the same thing, that makes it easier for us to all work together as a team.

And with this way of doing rounds we can do a lot of teaching. We can even teach about conflict resolution. We can discuss conflict resolution in a conference room, but we can really role model it in a room with a family. We can teach medical students and residents how to help a family in need. Selling to both members of my group and the residency program that the teaching is different and very valuable for residents and medical students. In the room I can teach about communication skills, about relationships, about having difficult conversations, about giving bad news. You'll have to do these every day. You can't teach this in normal rounds. It was the right thing to do. At first, our evaluations scores may have gone down because of the difference in teaching and rounding. But now they don't know anything different.

The tide changed when everybody realized it was here to stay—there was no going back. Then the nurses would meet us when we arrived on the floor. "Are you going to see my kids? I'm coming in." We have a great relationship with the nurses on this floor now. Now even aside from rounds, they'll stop us before we go in the patient room to give us a heads up if there's something that the family is concerned about or upset about. Before we would find out once we walked in the room and hardly ever BEFORE we walked in the room. Today a nurse gave me a heads up that the family hadn't heard back about some tests. So I wasn't blindsided. I called the two specialists and find out what was going on. When I went into the patient room I could anticipate the family's questions. It took 10 to 15 minutes before I went in the room, but it was worth its weight in gold. It would have taken more than that much time afterward if I didn't come in with the information. And families don't like it when they think we aren't talking to each other.

The most obvious benefits of family-centered rounds at Riley were accurate and timely communication, enabling patients to be discharged earlier in the day with fewer delays. Soon after the implementation of family-centered rounds at Riley, EEGs and MRIs were being completed in 1.73 hours relative to 2.15 hours prior to the rounds ($p = 0.001$). Moreover, 47% of patients were being discharged on the first shift compared with 40% of patients prior to family-centered rounds ($p = 0.004$). Other evidence suggests that timely movement of patients into and out of the hospital decreases the risk of adverse events. Saysana explained:

> All the evidence shows that the best thing for the patient is to get out of the hospital when they are ready to go, and for the patients who are waiting, the best thing is to get them in when they need to be admitted. Delays on either end increase the chance of adverse events. And if there's a care delay for patients coming from the ER [emergency room], they can end up in the ICU [intensive care unit].

In summary, family-centered rounds have improved throughput while reducing the risk of adverse events. More timely communication and faster discharges have also reduced waiting for patients and their families, both the waiting to be admitted on the front end, and the waiting to be discharged on the back end. On top of these benefits, patients and families experience fewer disconnects in information, thereby decreasing anxiety. How have these outcomes been achieved?

Success Factors

Although family-centered rounds are a relatively straightforward intervention, they are challenging to implement and sustain. Units in other medical centers have attempted implementation, and after initial enthusiasm the rounds often fade away, leaving participants cynical and resistant to further change efforts. According to a physician leader in an East Coast academic medical center:

> We implemented bedside rounds—we came up with clear protocols and roles. When everyone was there it worked well. The issue is getting everyone there at same time. You can't really schedule it. It's been hard to sustain—now it's falling apart and people are feeling cynical.

A key success factor at Riley has been an understanding that implementing the mechanics of family-centered rounds is not sufficient. It is also necessary to implement the relational dynamics to support the structure. In order to get timely, accurate, problem-solving communication to occur at the rounds, the leader must create a relational climate of mutual respect and shared knowledge, while connecting participants to their shared goals—the ultimate well-being of the patient and family. If these conditions are not met, staff will not attend, or will simply go through the motions. As Saysana explained:

> How we do the rounds is critical. We are really intentional about timing so everyone knows what time. We acknowledge each team member's role so they feel it's worth their time. Team members leave knowing the plan, how to follow up with the patient and how to answer the family's questions. And it opens up opportunities for us all to communicate outside the rounds.
>
> We introduce ourselves to the family, and we'll say something like—"May is your nurse and she's awesome—she's been a nurse longer than I've been a doctor." We say hello to the family and ask how are things going since I last saw you? We ask the nurses and pharmacists to participate during the rounds—and they do—then they know they are valuable. We show them that there's value to them being in the room. Then they feel more comfortable answering the family's questions afterward. If they are not in the room, then they can't answer the patient's questions as well—they feel bad.

Implementation is not a one-time effort. Professional cultures, professional training and scheduling practices continue to work against family-centered rounding so sustaining the rounds requires ongoing reinforcement.

> Everybody has to be reinforced. We say to the nurses, "We're going to see your patient—do you want to come with us?" We ask them things during the rounds so they don't feel like why do I have to be here? We want them to know their input is valued. They spend more time with the patient and family than any of the medical students, residents, or attending physicians. They have to see that together we are improving many of the processes for patients on that floor, including the admission and discharge processes.

Implementing Change: The Role of Relational Leadership

Clearly it is essential for leaders to model and reinforce relational dynamics within the rounds themselves. But what other roles do leaders play in the successful implementation of an innovation such as family-centered rounds? Dr. Saysana tells the story of family-centered rounds as emerging from a collective effort, but also described the role of both formal and informal leadership.

> When we started, I had no formal authority in my group of hospitalists or at Riley. I would say, "Come on! Why can't we do this? Why can't we try this?" The formal leader of our service supported it but really encouraged us to have a discussion about it. He did not tell us we had to do it, but instead he really supported us visiting another hospital and figuring out how we could do it. He's been gracious about it. He says I need to take credit for doing this. I usually don't. And the other medical services were not really interested in doing it. Then our ICU started it. All those who started it were not the chiefs, and they were not made to do it. My chair said it was a good idea, but he didn't make me do it. It was not formal, it just kind of spread on its own.

One characteristic of Saysana's informal leadership of the implementation effort was her respectful consideration of the resistance she faced from others. Rather than writing off resistance as "resistance to change" or ascribing it to selfish motives, she saw resistance as potentially containing valuable information about obstacles that deserved respectful consideration and that needed to be addressed. For example:

> The biggest pushback was from the person who is now my biggest advocate. He wanted to know, how are we going to do this? What if the medical student says in front of the family that the child might have cancer? Well they already do, I said, but you don't hear it. He still didn't want to do the rounds in the room, because he felt it would put the students on the spot.
>
> Fortuitously, there were new requirements in the pediatric residency curriculum that required pediatric residents to be observed interacting with patients. For me, that NEVER happened when I was training. Our pediatric residency program was struggling with how to do all of these direct observations and document this for every residents. I saw family-centered rounds as a

perfect opportunity. We put our observations directly into the residents' rotation evaluations. In the beginning some of the residents and students didn't really like it. They said it's going to be awkward, take too long. We really had to sell it to them. We told them, "We're going room to room and we're going to do ALL the work together." We will do all of the orders while we are in the room. We can call consults if we need to.

The nurses really wanted to do this. Typically we make all the big decisions and they have to do all the work. The pushback we got from the nurses was: "What about these families that want to take up all your time?" I said, "We can come back." But what we find is, we tell the families up front what's going on and then they don't have so many questions later.

Another barrier was the time issue. In a conference room with the residents, medical students, and the attending, we can round very fast on 10 kids. But you didn't really see them, so you're going to have to go back and see them again anyway. If the attending physician hasn't seen them before discussing them in the conference room, often the plans will change and more time will have to be spent communicating a new plan to all of the team. When we do family-centered rounds, I can see the patient while the discussion is taking place and the family can see how we process information and make decisions. Also, our administration said: "Why don't we give you laptops so you can look things up while you're doing rounds? We'll get you a cart and laptop and phones so you can have all these things on rounds with you." We became test pilots for new equipment. We are now seen as early adopters.

Leadership support from the hospital's top management also played a critical role, according to Saysana:

We had administrative support. Marilyn Cox is our chief nursing officer at Riley and she's a leader in safety and family and relationship-centered care. When she supports something, it happens, and I've watched her do it. She was very much a supporter and she wanted to make sure her nurses were participating. She was able to see that the nurses would do it.

Marilyn Cox sees relationship-centered care and mindful organizing as connected—also family-centered rounds, but less explicitly. For both, we're all on the same page. We are in the same room. You have to engage the nurse, ask them what concerns they have about this patient. You have to be intentional about doing it. Now nursing leaders tell their staff, "You are a big part of family-centered rounds because better communication improves safety." It's not just having the rounds that make the relationships good between doctors and nurses—it's HOW we do them. Other nurses come in from other units to watch. Marilyn talks to her managers a lot—tells them what's going on. She tells them family-centered rounds are a very important part of family-centered care, and that this is how we can help. We (hospitalists) also have about the best local relationships with the other physicians on our floor. The pain scores are best on our floor and the surgical floor due to our relationships with doctors and nurses.

The change to family-centered rounds needs physician leadership and buy-in. It doesn't take very MANY to buy in, but they need to be influencers in their group—they need to be at least informal leaders if not formal leaders. You have to have physicians with credibility in the group. Patients can be a catalyst, but the next step is to find that physician who will be the champion.

In addition to Saysana and her leaders within Riley Hospital, others in the health system were attentive to the relational dynamics involved in effective care delivery. The system had benefited over many years from cutting-edge research and practice on relationship-centered care by a team at the Regenstrief Institute under the leadership of Tom Inui, Debra Litzelman, and Richard Frankel.[19] Then in 2009, Gene Beyt was recruited as the Senior Vice President of Medical Quality to help lead Indiana University Health's quality improvement efforts. Beyt was recruited by the health system's board with a shared vision of the importance of relationships across all participants in the system—including patients—for achieving the highest levels of performance.

By 2011, much of the groundwork was in place, and a team of physician and nurse leaders had been formed. Dubbed the Relational Coordination Team, its members were united by the shared goal to improve the quality and efficiency of care by enhancing the relational climate in which care is delivered. Relational coordination was chosen as a broad umbrella concept that reflects many of the relational dynamics that drive the quality and efficiency of health care including relational climate, Appreciative Inquiry, and other related concepts.

Looking Forward

In early 2012, Gene Beyt and his colleagues in the Relational Coordination Team found themselves at a challenging decision point. Changing the relational climate for a large health-care system was a daunting task indeed, given the substantial obstacles posed by health-care professional identities, cultures, and training, particularly in academic systems. The imminent approval of the Patient Protection and Affordable Care Act by the US Supreme Court made their decision point even more challenging. On one hand, the new accountable care environment meant that the health system would be rewarded for improving the quality and efficiency of care, but on the other hand it meant that every initiative and budget item would be subject to intense scrutiny.

What was the potential for taking this basic intervention—family-centered rounds—and scaling it up to serve the system's entire 18-hospital system? Family-centered rounding within the system had thus far focused on pediatric units where families are a key component in the post-discharge success of the patient. However, families also play a critical role in the care of elders as well. In fact, the lack of spouse or family support leads to a number of post-discharge challenges, elevating the importance of discharge planning and strong receiving agencies in the community. Could family-centered rounds serve as an effective point of entry for other changes to occur over time? What supports would be needed to ensure the sustained success of this intervention, based on the subtle relational dynamics that characterized its successful implementation at Riley Hospital for Children?

Discussion

This case study offers a useful example of relational leadership. The faculty and staff at Riley were not mandated to implement family-centered rounds; rather, they were engaged in making a site visit and assessing the feasibility. When they encountered objections from colleagues, they listened deeply. They heard and legitimated the fears and concerns about family-centered rounds and they learned enough about their colleagues' work processes that they were able to reframe this new form of rounding as a solution to other problems (e.g., saving time by not having to go back and revisit each patient later in the day). Thinking outside of the silo of the patient care unit to recognize larger organizational needs, they gained critical momentum by framing family-centered rounds as a solution to a new educational accreditation requirement for direct observation of students' interactions with patients and families. In these and other ways, the leadership process by which the rounds were introduced involved fostering shared goals; learning more about each other's work processes, needs and concerns, thus developing shared knowledge; and both demonstrating and deepening respect—the foundations of relational leadership.

The Relational Model of Organizational Change, shown in Figure 6.2, offers further insights into this case study of relational leadership. This model reflects research that shows relational processes drive critical outcomes including quality, efficiency, and the well-being of participants.

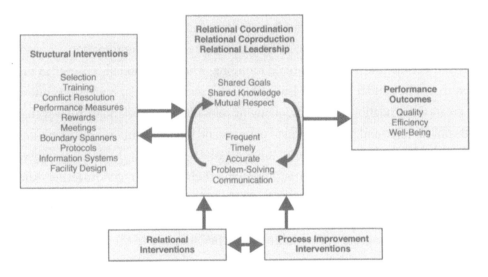

FIGURE 6.2 Relational Model of Organizational Change

The model also addresses the question—which kinds of interventions are effective in transforming relational processes from the highly fragmented dynamics that we often observe in traditional organizations, into the cohesive relational dynamics that we observe in high-performing, nimble organizations? Based on the work of Gittell, Edmondson, and Schein,[1] the Relational Model of Organizational Change identifies three components of an effective, sustainable transformational effort: (1) relational interventions, such as cultural islands or conversations of interdependence or relational mapping, to create new kinds of dynamics and conversations; (2) process improvement interventions such as lean or quality management to bring participants together to explore the nature of their work and to create a context for the relational intervention; and (3) structural interventions in everyday organizational practices such as hiring, training, performance measurement, rewards, conflict resolution, information systems, and so on, to create cross-cutting structures that reinforce and sustain the new ways of working together.

Examined through the lens of this model, we can see that family-centered rounding is both a process improvement and a relational intervention. As a work process, it provides a setting in which the diverse members of the care team (including patients and families) can coordinate their work more effectively. Bringing everyone together in one place facilitates timely and accurate communication and facilitates the integration of their various unique perspectives and needs to create shared goals and a shared, more holistic understanding of the patient's needs and care plan. Family-centered rounding is a process improvement intervention that facilitates the development of relational coordination.

At the same time family-centered rounding, when intentionally enacted in the way that is was under Saysana's leadership, also serves as a relational intervention. It creates new relational patterns, changing roles and power relations in a way that lifts up the voice and participation of patients and family members and distributes information, power, and authority more evenly. It allows all the team members to understand one another better, improving their ability to work together. And it offers everyone a new and better experience of teamwork, thus raising their expectations for what teamwork could and should look like in the future. They might hold one another accountable to a higher standard in the future given the recognition that the old way no longer suffices.

We can also understand family-centered rounding through the lens of Complex Responsive Processes of Relating, a recently developed theory of human interaction that combines principles from social constructionism and complexity. According to this theory, the team members are creating and maintaining knowledge, including patterns of thinking, in the course of their conversations about the patient's situation and needs.[20] The emergence of new ideas in their conversation—the heart of innovation and adaptability—requires both diversity and responsiveness.[11] Family-centered rounds are a vehicle for diversity; team members encounter one another's different perspectives. To the extent that they listen responsively to one another, demonstrating openness and curiosity, their preexisting patterns of thinking are disturbed. New ideas emerge which can grow to become new integrative ways of thinking that are more robust and comprehensive.

The same behavior supports communication that is conducive to innovation, fostering responsiveness and the expression of diversity, particularly mutual respect, frequency, timeliness, and problem solving without blaming. Responsiveness also corresponds with humble inquiry, which we considered earlier in this chapter. Family-centered rounds may work as a trigger for broader organizational changes by providing participants with daily opportunities to practice reciprocal forms of interrelating such as relational leadership, relational coordination, and relational coproduction, thereby creating new or deeper relationships between workers and managers, workers and workers, and workers and customers, that tend to be replicated throughout the organization, transforming the way care is delivered.

However, for the sustainability of these new relational dynamics, the Relational Model of Organizational Change tells us that other changes are needed. In particular, the infrastructure of the organization—selection, training, conflict resolution, performance measurement, rewards, and so forth—will likely need to be redesigned to embed the new relational patterns into participant roles, going beyond the individuals themselves. In recent work, Gittell and Douglass[6] explore in depth these macrostructures and how they embed reciprocal relationships into roles in depth.

Conclusion

The story of family-centered rounding at Riley Hospital for Children offers fine examples of all three forms of reciprocal interrelating. *Relational coproduction* takes place as patients, family members, and clinicians communicate in a frequent and timely manner to share their different perspectives and develop shared understanding and shared goals for care. *Relational coordination* is similarly present in the exchange and collaboration between physicians, nurses, students, pharmacists, and all the other professionals on the care team. These highly relational patterns of interaction involving patients and staff members could only be introduced and sustained by a process that embodied and reinforced the same values, *relational leadership*. As these team members experience a work environment of respect and responsiveness, it's easier for them to turn toward patients, family members, and their colleagues and treat them the same way.

We have also seen that the aligned action and broader understanding that comes from frequent, timely, and respectful interactions reduces waste and error, streamlines care, and enhances satisfaction of patients and staff alike. Family-centered rounding offers us yet another example of how relationships matter, another component of wisdom leadership.

References

1. Gittell JH, Edmondson A, Schein E. Learning to coordinate: a relational model of organizational change. *Proceedings of the Academy of Management.* 2011 August 12–16; San Antonio, TX. Academy of Management Publishing.
2. Tresolini C. Health professions education and relationship-centered care. *Report of the Pew-Fetzer Task Force on Advancing Psychosocial Education.* San Francisco, CA: Pew Health Commission; 1994.
3. Mitchell P, Wynia M, Golden R, *et al. Core Principles and Values of Effective Team-based Health Care* [discussion paper]. Washington, DC: Institute of Medicine; 2012. Available at: www.iom.edu/tbc (accessed October 8, 2012)
4. Ancona D, Bresman H. *X-teams: how to build teams that lead, innovate and succeed.* Boston, MA: Harvard Business School Publishing; 2007.
5. Carson JB, Tesluk PE, Marrone JA. Shared leadership in teams: an investigation of antecedent conditions and performance. *Acad Manage J.* 2007; **50**(5): 1217–34.
6. Gittell JH, Douglass A. Relational bureaucracy: structuring reciprocal relationships into roles. *Acad Manage Rev.* 2012; **37**(4): 709–54.
7. Lipman-Blumen, J. Connective leadership: female leadership styles in the 21st century workplace. *Sociol Perspect.* 1992; **35**(1): 183–203.
8. Gilligan C. *In a Different Voice: psychological theory and women's development.* Cambridge, MA: Harvard University Press; 1982.
9. Fletcher JK. Leadership, power, and positive relationships. In: Dutton JE, Ragins BR, editors. *Exploring Positive Relationships at Work: building a theoretical and research foundation.* New York, NY: Psychology Press; 2007. pp. 347–71.
10. Schein E. *Helping: how to offer, give and receive help.* San Francisco: Berrett-Koehler; 2011.
11. Suchman AL. A new theoretical foundation for relationship-centered care. *J Gen Intern Med.* 2006; **21**: S40–4.
12. Adler PS, Kwon S, Heckscher C. Professional work: the emergence of collaborative community. *Organ Sci.* 2008; **19**: 359–76.
13. Douglass A, Gittell JH. Transforming professionalism: relational bureaucracy and parent-teacher partnerships in child care settings. *J Child Res.* 2012; **10**(3): 267–81.
14. Sisterhen LL, Blaszak RT, Woods MB, *et al.* Defining family-centered rounds. *Teach Learn Med.* 2007; **19**(3): 319–22.

15. Uhlig PN, Brown J, Nason AK, *et al.* John M. Eisenberg Patient Safety Awards. System Innovation: Concord Hospital. *Jt Comm J Qual Improv.* 2002; **28**(12): 666–72.

16. Muething SE, Kotagal UR, Schoettker PJ, *et al.* Family-centered bedside rounds: a new approach to patient care and teaching. *Pediatrics.* 2007; **119**: 829–32.

17. Kuzin JK, Yborra JG, Taylor MD. Family-member presence during interventions in the intensive care unit: perceptions of pediatric cardiac intensive care providers. *Pediatrics.* 2007; **120**: 895–901.

18. Davidson JE, Powers K, Hedayat KM, *et al.* Clinical practice guidelines for support of the family in the patient-centered intensive care unit: American College of Critical Care Medicine Task Force 2004–2005. *Crit Care Med.* 2007; **35**(2): 605–22.

19. Williamson P, Baldwin DC, Cottingham AH, *et al.* Transforming the professional culture of a medical school from the inside out. In: Suchman AL, Sluyter D, Williamson P, editors. *Leading Change in Healthcare: transforming organizations with complexity, positive psychology and relationship-centered care.* London: Radcliffe; 2011.

20. Stacey R. *Complex Responsive Processes in Organizations: learning and knowledge creation.* New York, NY: Routledge; 2001.

Finding Our Positive Emotion

WILEY SOUBA, IN CHAPTER 10, WILL TALK ABOUT LEADERSHIP AS A "WAY of being" that requires us to be able to see things differently in order to open up opportunities for right action and for leading from what he calls our natural self-expression. Particularly in situations of constraint, situations that seem hopelessly limited, leaders who stand out are leaders who can reframe the conversation, from deficit to opportunity. Leaders like this bring out the best in people, and help them to do things they never thought possible. Suddenly insurmountable problems become keys to success, and unresolvable conflicts become the foundation of strong positive relationships.

The story that follows exemplifies how both patients/families and providers can inspire one another and bring out one another's best selves, doing the seemingly impossible with grace. The subsequent chapter on positivity reveals some of the science behind this process of reframing and focused attention on finding our best selves, and it describes ways to foster this in our academic health science center. Again, like reflection and compassion, bringing out the best in one another is a practice, a discipline, not a one-time decision. Like exercise, it gets easier and more reliable with practice.

A Story: Holy Moments

Jim Ogan

I suspect holy moments are present all around us all the time. Some are more memorable than others of course, but I suspect they are always there. Like the air when it becomes a breeze, or a cloud when it becomes fog, holy moments happen and we are already there, or not. We can choose to notice the breeze as it gently grazes our face, the wind messing up our hair, a gust threatening a hat's safety, or we can plow along, head down, headstrong, intent and intense about getting on with life's business.

And so it goes with patients. We can move from one to the next politely and efficiently doing the business of doctoring, nursing. And isn't it the same with the young woman at the checkout, or with the teller at the bank? I'm told that people don't go into the bank much anymore. Apparently, most of us don't have the need to chat about the weather, or baseball while completing our transactions.

I suspect a sense of awe and wonder would invade our preoccupation with expertise and efficiency more often if we allowed for its spontaneity. If we approached our work and our lives with a willingness to be surprised by the unexpected, we might be delighted with an abundance of holy moments and awe.

As a pediatrician, I frequently have the opportunity to be present at the birth of a newborn baby. I am called to the deliveries that may pose a hazardous entry into life for the little ones. To be sure, it can be quite tense standing by, waiting for the birth of a newborn whose heart rate has dipped perilously low, or whose bowels have relinquished their meconium into the normally clear amniotic fluid, or, God forbid, the placenta begins to hemorrhage. I have found this kind of mischief to get the catecholamines flowing, prepping me for what is to come.

Still, most of these deliveries turn out just fine. A baby emerges and offers a lusty cry for all the world to hear. And at that moment you may be surprised to learn that there are often tears. I routinely see the dads bashfully dabbing the wetness from their eyes, while gently kissing the noble new mother's sweat soaked head. And, depending on how harrowing the birth, there can be tears of relief that spontane-ously fill the eyes of even the most experienced nurse or doctor. Then again, tears in the delivery room are not that unusual.

Perhaps it is simply the miracle of birth, which never gets old. The primal drama of pushing and grunting and sweating and groaning a baby into the world can never become completely routine, or can it? When I'm called for a potential crisis, and stand ready to address any emergency that might ruin a happy ending, the routine is tense and the delight of a lusty cry is always a welcome miracle. Some might say an ordinary miracle.

Last year, Charlie arrived about 6 weeks prematurely. His circumstance had been well documented with a dozen prenatal ultrasounds, so everyone knew well in advance that Charlie's skull would be enormous, and his arms and legs would be abnormally short. We suspected that his thorax would be too small for his lungs to grow big enough to support life. Everyone was ready for Charlie's birth, his neonatal intensive care unit (NICU) stay, and his likely early demise. He was to be one of only five other children alive with thanatophoric dysplasia, type I.

Indeed, Charlie's birth may have been the most routine part of his entire life. The first 3 months in the NICU were a constant cascade of near-death plunges into apnea and bradycardia, the likes of which earned him the nickname of eggplant man because of the purple hue that became him in his near-death events.

Still, the NICU works miracles every day and Charlie graduated with his vent and his gastrostomy tube to Kluge Children's Rehabilitation Center in Charlottesville, Virginia, for another month before finally making it home on Valentine's Day.

In pediatrics we are all about tracking and assessing growth and development. As anyone who works with children knows well, there are norms and scales for every developmental domain: social, intellectual, fine motor, gross motor. Pediatricians are the geeks of developmental assessment. We also enjoy monitoring growth by plotting heights and weights on tidy, color-coded curves. Parents enjoy it too, chuckling over a head circumference at the ninety-fifth percentile, or a weight that is off the curve. Generally, parents find comfort in hearing that their babies are meeting predictable milestones: smiling at 6 weeks, opening their hands by 3 months, crawling by 9 months, and having 18 words at 18 months. These are the ordinary, delightful, miracles of every well child visit.

But then there's Charlie, never to grow or sit or talk in any typically measurable or ordinary way. His head is far too big for him to safely sit without major support. His tracheostomy and continuous mechanical ventilation impede speech. His arms have only recently become long enough and strong enough for him to touch his own face, and he cannot yet scratch his own nose.

Still, nearing 18 months old, he eats solid food, drinks from a cup, and waves bye-bye to me as I leave. Charlie enjoys watching his brothers and his sister play and smiles at them, happy with their exploits and attention.

Last month, I joined all of Charlie's therapists and nurses for a team meeting in his home. We gathered to discuss his progress and our goals and plans for the coming months. The engineers were present to refit his stroller that must accommodate his heavy head and his ventilator so he might be more mobile with the family. We discussed feeding and language with occupational, and speech, therapists. We contemplated molds and braces with the physical therapist to help with increased strength and weight bearing on his tenuous spine and tiny, weak legs. Near the end, Charlie's mom, Erin, lay him down on an activity mat in the middle of the room for everyone to see his newest skill. We all gathered around to coax and encourage and cheer him as he struggled mightily to *roll over*!

Standing there looking on with the others, I remember thinking to myself:

> Oh Charlie, can you really hope to do this ordinary, yet complex gross motor task of a 5- or 6-month-old baby? You are attached to a mechanical ventilator. You have tiny arms and legs with poor muscle tone, and a giant head you have no way of lifting on your own. And yet, there you are in front of me, a beaming smile, heaving to and fro a little bit at a time, working up the momentum, like I remember trying to do in a canoe in the middle of the lake, rocking and rocking until finally, *wow*, Charlie, there you are face down on the mat.

Of course Charlie's crowd went wild, whooping and hollering, followed abruptly with real concern for his safety, now being upside down, on top of the ventilator tubing, with no apparent way to get righted. Instinctively we leaned in to help. Erin smiled proudly and gently dispelled our desire to rescue. Instead, she encouraged Charlie to roll back over on his own, adding that he hadn't quite mastered this, but eventually she knew he would. So, just as abruptly, we got back to being Charlie's adoring fans, and wouldn't you know, he heaved and rocked and wiggled his way right back over, onto his back? And don't you know when he did, he looked up at each one of us in the circle with *the most, amazing, satisfied smile* you will ever see. Man oh man, don't you know that was one holy moment indeed.

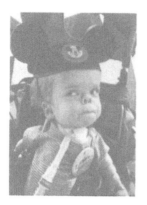 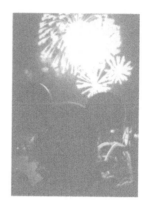

In early 2013, Charlie took the "trip of a lifetime" with his family to Disney World, ventilator and all. Charlie's family is delighted to share these photos with you.

7

Finding Our Positive Emotion

Julie Haizlip and Margaret Plews-Ogan

Positivity transforms us for the better . . ..

*By opening our hearts and minds, positive emotions allow us to discover
and build new skills, new ties, new knowledge and new ways of being.*

—Barbara Fredrickson[1]

POSITIVITY IN HEALTH CARE IS NOT A NEW CONCEPT. MANY SCIENTISTS and casual observers have posited that optimism and positivity have the potential to improve health.[2] Optimism has been found to have a protective effect against the development of cardiovascular disease.[3] A sense of well-being has been demonstrated to positively affect survival in renal failure and HIV.[3] And, there has been considerable research looking at the effect of positivity on survival in cancer.[4] Other investigators suggest that positive emotion may even have a favorable impact on the duration and severity of the common cold![5,6] As health-care professionals, we are intrigued by how our patients and their health might be affected by their mood and outlook. Much less consideration has been given to the idea that mood might also affect health-care providers and the organizations in which they work.

A tremendous body of literature suggests that negativity influences many domains of human existence.[7] Aspects of our lives from memory to relationships are profoundly altered by negative experiences. Much thought has been given to stress and burnout in health-care professionals, but the realm of the effect of "in the moment" emotion on the performance of health-care professionals remains largely unexplored. Perhaps, much the way that we seem to expect that our determination and commitment trumps routine illness and sleep deprivation, we expect that our intellect and professionalism can buffer us from our own emotional experience. Sir William Osler[8,9] often noted the importance of the heart and the mind as a therapeutic tool in doctoring. In an 1899 address at the Albany Medical College he warned young physicians, "be careful as you get into practice to cultivate equally well your hearts and your heads."[8] Yet in a seemingly contradictory statement, Osler suggested that "imperturbability"[9] was the foremost quality of a physician. He further described this trait as "coolness and presence of mind under all circumstances, calmness amid storm, clearness of judgment in moments of grave peril."[9] If one possesses imperturbability as well as experience and knowledge, Osler asserted, "No eventuality can disturb the mental equilibrium of the physician."[9] When one achieves this "aequanimitas," it is possible to put the needs of the patient first and foremost and not be distracted by one's own experience. It appears that modern medical culture has interpreted aequanimitas to mean that the emotions of a provider are to be stifled rather than acknowledged, and that we have perhaps forgotten Osler's admonition to "cultivate equally well your hearts and your heads."[8] Recently, a colleague described caring for a critically ill patient who was similar in age to his own daughter and the emotion it stirred in him. He quickly followed this with a statement explaining how he immediately stored those thoughts away in his "professional closet" so that he could provide the necessary care to the patient and her family.

There is increasing awareness that despite our efforts to achieve aequanimitas as health-care professionals we are indeed influenced by our interactions with patients and colleagues.[10] We react to the time pressures and scheduling challenges, the frustrations with changing technologies and realities of documentation and pre-authorization. Despite our best efforts, our performance and the resulting care of our patients is affected. This chapter explores how intentional positivity can create change in our everyday activities in academic health-care institutions. Positivity favorably impacts individuals as well as the performance of teams, and can thereby improve the care we provide to those we serve.

The World We Live In and How We Got Here

In health care, we spend a lot of time thinking about what is wrong. In pathophysiology, we focus on what happens when something in the body goes awry. Our visits with patients often begin with the "Chief Complaint." We have been taught to rule out the worst-case scenario so that we don't miss a critical situation and then we plan how to respond if the patient's condition deteriorates.[11] We share bad news or troubling diagnoses with patients and families. At times, we bear witness with a family as their loved one dies. In academic settings, we experience these things firsthand, and also have them reinforced time and time again as we educate the next generations of physicians, nurses, and other health professionals. The tradition of "pimping" students to reveal what they have failed to memorize reinforces what students lack rather than building on what they know or have done well. This approach creates vigilance for, and an expectation of, failure. Those who "survive" this approach to training often feel justified, as a rite of passage, to perpetuate the ritual in successive generations of trainees.

All the time we spend intentionally focusing on the negative reinforces an evolutionary construct known as the negativity bias. The negativity bias describes the well-evidenced concept that we are more greatly influenced by negative experiences than by positive ones. Presumably, those who have had a keen eye toward threat and danger have had a survival advantage as we have evolved. Scientists have demonstrated that the negativity bias affects us across a broad range of the human experience.[8,12] For example, psychologists have found that the potential for negative repercussions leads to faster and more permanent learning than the promise of reward. We spend much more effort and thought trying to make sense of negative events and experiences than we do considering pleasant ones. Our relationships are profoundly impacted by negative interactions; a single traumatic encounter can supplant many positive ones and shape future communications. These and other findings suggest that our reactions to negativity are instinctive and have long-lasting ramifications. It is worth considering that these basic reactions affect our work in health care—especially when our educational processes reinforce these messages multiple times each day. By the very nature of what we do, health-care professionals spend a tremendous amount of time focusing on the negative aspects of people's lives.[13] Over time, we become conditioned and find coping mechanisms to deal with the most challenging of these experiences. Chronically faced with the physical, mental, and emotional demands of providing health care, many physicians and nurses become burned out.[14-17] Stress is not limited to interactions with patients and family members. It also occurs in encounters with one another. Differing opinions and high-stakes circumstances can lead to heated exchanges. Despite a shared interest in providing the best care for patients, these encounters can profoundly damage working relationships.[18] Our formal education process includes morbidity and mortality reviews that fully and carefully evaluate bad outcomes. Perhaps most devastating, the majority of us will be make medical errors. In this situation, we spend many hours recreating the situation, questioning our judgment, suffering disproportionately because we have hurt another human being, analyzing the breakdowns in the system, and fearing the potential ramifications.[19,20] Ultimately, we find ourselves instinctively identifying the negative possibilities in everything around us—our patients, our colleagues, the system, and ourselves. These thoughts impact everything from our relationships with others to the way we function in teams and even our ability to create strategic plans.

Anthropologists and sociologists teach us that cultures are formed by the collective thoughts and traditions of the members of the group; the culture of academic medicine has become one that is grounded in negativity. This is one possible explanation for why so many physicians express dissatisfaction with their experiences in academic medicine.[21] It might offer some insight into the high incidence of alcohol and drug dependence in physicians. This inherent bias toward the negative and its serial reinforcement in medical education may also contribute to depression and suicide rates among health-care professionals that are much higher than the general population.[22,23]

Our Experience

During a particularly difficult time in the recent past at the University of Virginia School of Medicine, David Leach, MD—then president of the Accreditation Council for Graduate Medical Education—suggested that we use Appreciative Inquiry (AI)[24] to help our faculty reconnect with the meaning of our work and to remember why we chose a career in academic medicine. The process of AI begins with finding the best in an organization through narrative accounts of times that things went well. With the help of Rich Frankel, PhD, from Indiana University, we held a retreat with representation from many of the academic departments. When asked to reflect on a time in academic medicine that was meaningful to them, faculty members told beautiful stories about influential connections with their students and patients, productive collaborations and scientific innovations. We heard narratives describing remarkable empathy and compassion and there was an expression of awe and privilege around our everyday experience.[25]

The following story is from the retreat.

As residents we get very busy and stressed out and sometimes forget that we can make a difference in somebody's life. I was helping to take care of a 14-year-old girl with a recent diagnosis of AML [acute myeloid leukemia]. It felt like every time I walked into this girl's room she was upset with me. I'd say something stupid like, "Oh, is your hair starting to fall out?" and she'd cry. Or I'd ask, "Is that rash itchy?" and she said, "Of course it is, are you stupid?"

She always wanted to know when one of the attendings would be in, and why did I have to examine her in addition to Dr. W, or Dr. D? She really didn't want to have anything to do with me, but every day I came in and examined her and got to know her a little bit. One morning, just as I was about to pre-round, I heard an overhead page for the on-call resident to a room number that was hers. A bunch of people started to run, but I beat them there.

She was sitting up in bed, her sats (oxygen saturation measures) were down in the low 80s, her blood pressure was low, her heart rate was up, and she looked

> at me with the most grave face I have ever seen. Platelets were infusing. We stopped the platelets, gave saline, watched her vitals, and over the course of about 10 minutes she was looking much better.
>
> I said, "OK, I'm going to go out and call the blood bank and call Dr. D. so that she can come in and make sure everything is OK," but the patient reached out her hand, touched me on the elbow, and said, "Don't go." And so I didn't. Maybe it was just seeing my face every day; there was something comforting about my presence in the room when she was scared, when she thought she was dying. After the first few minutes I had no medical purpose for being in the room, but she wanted me there. I mean, how moving is that? . . . that our job lets us affect somebody that way?

Participants left the retreat feeling energized and reconnected to one another and to the meaning in their work as teachers and learners. It wasn't long before several faculty members approached us asking to create a similar experience for the members of their division, department, or practice setting. This type of work was clearly resonating.

Ultimately, we have formed an infrastructure (the University of Virginia [UVA] Center for Appreciative Practice) that allows us to continue working with groups from our health system to explore what is working well and to help them create common visions of the future that aspire to that ideal. Several groups have made remarkable changes that have affected employee engagement and patient satisfaction.[26] Interestingly, despite these results and the fact that people generally enjoy working with us, we do still meet resistance when we introduce our positive approach. In our scientifically focused community, it is difficult to sell the idea that a process that is enjoyable and creates positive emotion can actually generate desired change. This skepticism led us to explore the evidence for the use of positivity in more depth.

Evidence for the Use of Positivity

If one asks if there is scientific evidence demonstrating that positivity can change the culture in academic health care, the answer is not exactly. However, there is substantial data that positivity can impact many aspects of our work, including individual and team functioning, that factor into our daily experiences.

Representative samples of the many studies that could apply to academic medicine and health science centers are presented here.

Positivity and the Individual

Martin Seligman and his colleagues at the University of Pennsylvania have done remarkable work that demonstrates how positivity can affect individuals. In 2005, they published a randomized, controlled trial looking at a number of potential positive interventions and their effect on individual happiness and depression.[27] In this study of 577 adults, participants were assigned one of six tasks—five of which were postulated to potentially improve happiness, and one that was a control condition. The interventions included (1) keeping a diary of early childhood memories (control), (2) writing and delivering a letter of gratitude, (3) keeping a diary of three things that went well each day, (4) writing and reviewing a reflection of when you were at your best, (5) identifying one's signature strengths, and (6) using one's signature strengths in a new way. Each participant engaged in his or her assigned activity for 1 week. The gratitude visit resulted in an immediate significant increase in happiness and decrease in depression that lasted at least one month. The two exercises that entailed using one's signature strengths and keeping a diary of three good things a day for a single week each demonstrated an immediate and sustained decrease in depression and increased happiness at 1-, 3-, and 6-month measurements.

Barbara Fredrickson[1] has also studied the impact of positivity on individuals. In longitudinal studies of a large group of university students, she and Thomas Joiner found that those students with more positivity in their lives were more able to cope with adversity and to find solutions to their challenges. Additionally, the students with greater positivity were more apt to find solutions that, in turn, reinforced their outlook leading to personal growth and increased trust.[1]

Plews-Ogan *et al.*[28] have studied how people respond positively to adversity. They recently completed a study on physicians who had made a serious medical error. They found that the physicians who did well after this difficult experience (classified by the researchers blinded to the questionnaire results as wisdom exemplars) scored higher in positive emotions, including gratitude and positive emotions on the Neuroticism-Extroversion-Openness (NEO) personality inventory.[29,30]

Positivity and Education

Following his work on the effects of positivity on the individual, Seligman[3] received a grant to investigate whether embedding personal strength assessments, gratitude, and other positive interventions would make a difference in a cohort of 347 high school students. In this study, elements of positivity and strength-spotting were incorporated into the language arts curriculum for half of the students, while the other half continued in the standard curriculum. The goals of the "treatment" curriculum included promoting resilience, positive emotion and positive social relationships. The students identified their signature strengths and increased the use of these strengths in their daily lives. Questionnaires were administered to students, their parents, and "blinded" teachers before and after the study period and for 2 additional years. The results were compelling. Students who were enrolled in the curriculum including positivity were found to have greater curiosity, creativity, and love of learning. They achieved higher grades in language arts for the duration of the study through eleventh grade. The students reported more enjoyment and engagement in school. Teachers and parents reported improved social skills such as empathy, cooperation, self-control, and assertiveness.

Positivity in Medical Diagnostic Reasoning and other Complex Decision-Making Contexts

Two very interesting studies have been undertaken that look at diagnostic reasoning in medicine. The first was a study of volunteer medical students who were observed as they reasoned through a series of six patient care scenarios to determine which were most likely to represent a diagnosis of lung cancer. Immediately prior to the task, each of the students completed a brief word puzzle. Half were praised on their performance to induce positive affect and half completed the task with no feedback. The students who had the induced positive mood demonstrated more efficient problem solving by reaching the correct answers more quickly and with greater organization than their peers who were not praised. Interestingly, they spent an equivalent amount of time as controls because they went beyond the scope of the task—trying to establish diagnoses for the other patients as well.[31]

Similarly, 44 internists were enrolled in an observational study focused on their clinical reasoning as they engaged in a simulated case of a patient with chronic active hepatitis. As with the student study, a positive affect was induced in half of the study subjects. This was achieved with a simple note thanking the subject for participating and a small bag of candy. The internists who received the candy more quickly identified that the patient had liver disease yet did not prematurely anchor on the diagnosis. They continued to interpret all additional data that was presented and use it to further refine their clinical impression.[32]

Studies in other populations have evaluated the effect of positivity in complex decision making. In each of these investigations, positive affect was induced using a fairly minimal stimulus that would be of similar magnitude to an everyday experience (i.e., being told thank you, receiving a small bag of candy, watching a funny movie clip). This work has consistently shown that positive affect enhances problem solving and decision making. It also demonstrated that cognitive processes are more flexible, creative and innovative without sacrificing thoroughness and efficiency. Additionally, positivity was found to foster intrinsic motivation and stimulate interest in appealing tasks while preserving responsible work behavior.[33–35]

Positivity and Team Functioning

Studies looking at the impact of positive affect have also demonstrated enhanced characteristics that could improve team functioning such as increased helping behaviors, generosity, and interpersonal understanding. Losada and Heaphy[36] performed a fascinating study aimed at characterizing interactions between team members in high-, medium-, and low-functioning teams. Teams were classified based on standard business metrics including profitability, 360-degree evaluations and customer satisfaction. When Losada and Heaphy's[36] researchers observed team meetings, they identified and quantified elements of the conversations. One variable that they specifically examined was the frequency of positive and negative comments. The researchers found that the quantity of positive comments was much greater in the high-functioning teams, with a positive to negative ratio of 5.6:1. In contrast, the medium- and low-functioning teams had ratios of 1.8:1 and 0.36:1 respectively. The cause and effect relationship is unclear; do people speak to each other more favorably because it is a high-functioning team or is it a high-functioning team because the members communicate positively? While further research will be needed, particularly in the evolving sciences around relational coordination as noted in Chapter 6, it is clear that there is an association between positive communication styles and the successful performance of a team. Another variable Losada and Heaphy's[36] group measured was presence of inquiry and self-advocacy. Here they found that the high-performing teams were much more likely to explore one another's ideas and comments through inquiry whereas the lower-functioning teams spent much more time advocating for their point of view.

Medical teams may be best characterized as self-managing groups. Self-managing groups are characterized by a high degree of autonomy and control over their tasks. These groups have the flexibility to manage their own schedules and allocation of work. They are responsible for the quality of their work and are empowered to solve interpersonal conflicts among themselves. The leadership of these groups is often determined by which member has the greatest expertise about a particular issue and roles may change accordingly. Sy *et al.*[37] were interested in how the mood of the leader of a self-managing group affected the rest of the team. In their experimental design, the leaders of self-managing groups were randomly assigned to watch a video clip designed to induce either a positive or a negative mood in the leader. The groups were then monitored as they each performed the same task. This experiment demonstrated that the mood of the leader affected both the moods of the individual team members and the affective tone of the group. Leaders with an induced positive mood had a positive influence on the members of the team and the overall team affect. The study also demonstrated that while the teams with a leader in a negative mood produced greater effort, the teams with a positive leader had better team coordination. The net effect was that there was no difference found in overall task performance. In other words, there is nothing lost in a team that functions positively and enjoys its work. This study did not look at long-term outcomes and more research will be needed to determine whether there are additional benefits to organizing and working in a context ruled by negative or positive affect.

Positivity in Quality Improvement

Quality improvement is another arena in which early research suggests that positivity may play a unique and important role. Traditionally, quality programs have focused on what is *not* working in health systems, and developed "fixes" to address these deficits. This approach has obvious value, but it also has drawbacks. As many involved in quality will acknowledge, being constantly immersed in what is wrong can be demoralizing and exhausting. Although we have been working for years to solve quality problems, many continue unabated. Tackling these problems requires energy and creativity. Often our "solutions" fail because we lack a clear understanding of the context-dependent nature of effective solutions.

Positive Deviance (PD) and AI, both positive approaches to change, take a different stance. A fundamental principle in both PD and AI is that, "In every community there are certain individuals whose uncommon practices and behaviors enable them to find better solutions to problems than their neighbors who have access to the same resources."[38] PD has its roots in public health nutrition, specifically work by Tufts University nutrition professor Marion Zeitlin in the 1980s as she explored why some children in resource poor households did better than others with the same resource limitations.[39] In 1990 Monique and Jerry Sternin, familiar with Zeitlin's work, were tasked with addressing the severe and persistent problem of malnutrition in Vietnam. The Sternins decided to take a different approach to this situation than had ever been tried before. After arriving in the community and assessing the degree of malnutrition they were facing, they posed the question: "Are there any children who, despite these scarce resources, are thriving?" Well, *yes*, was the answer. So they went to see those families to discover what they were doing that made them successful. What the positive deviant families were doing was collecting tiny shrimp and crabs from the rice fields and adding them to their children's meals. They also added greens of local sweet potato plants to their children's food, fed them more often (three to four times per day rather than the traditional two times a day), washed their children's hands before they ate and actively fed them rather than simply putting the food in front of them.[38] With this local successful experience to build on, the Sternins developed a process to engage other mothers in the community with these successful mothers to learn and practice the essential new behaviors in four "intervention" villages. Results after two years were astonishing. Malnutrition decreased by 85% in the intervention PD communities. The PD intervention was subsequently adopted as a nationwide program. Follow-up studies confirmed those successive generations of Vietnamese children in the PD program villages were well nourished.[40]

PD, which will be discussed in detail in Chapter 8, is now being used in quality improvement initiatives across the country. Singhal *et al.*[38] described a national collaborative using positive deviance to reduce methicillin-resistant *Staphylococcus aureus* infections in hospitals. Successes at Waterbury Hospital in Connecticut, the VA Pittsburgh Health Care system, Albert Einstein and the Billings Clinic have also caught people's attention. The network of hospitals now using positive deviance techniques to prevent health care associated infections has expanded to 59 institutions.[38]

AI is another positive change approach that closely parallels the positive deviance approach. AI begins a change process with the same assumption: that someone, somewhere in the organization is performing well. Find those people, learn what works, and grow it up. AI has been used to improve handoff of care in residency training and in nursing.[41] In the situation of handoff of care, best practice had not yet been clearly defined and AI was used as a technique to "discover" best practice. AI and PD approaches can therefore be used to "discover" and define best practices when they are not known, to infuse positivity and energy into a quality improvement process, and to refine or adapt a known best practice (such as hand washing) to a particular environment to give it the best chance of success.

Summary of positivity research

To summarize, gratitude and a positive perspective increase individual happiness and decrease depression.[27] Positivity engages students and enhances school performance and social skills.[27] Complex decision making including medical diagnostic reasoning improves and is more creative in those with an induced positive affect. There is an association between positive communication and enhanced team performance,[36] and a leader's affect can influence group mood and team dynamics.[37] Finally, positive approaches to change (PD and AI) can be successfully applied to quality improvement. While only a few of these studies specifically involve academic medicine, one could infer that positivity offers tremendous potential to help us create the culture we desire.

Making Appreciative Inquiry Work

As we know, one mechanism that can instill positivity is AI. AI is an organizational change methodology that begins with the assumption that in every organization, there are people, teams, practices, and processes that are doing things well.[24] The process of AI is fundamentally grounded in valuing what is good and successful and inquiring into those successes to lead to further success. Using its

"4-D cycle," AI *discovers* the best of what is (the positive core), *dreams* about the ideal future, *designs* specific strategies to move the organization from where it is to where it wants to be, and *delivers* that goal. The process uses unconditionally positive questions that direct the responder to talk about highpoint experiences. For example, asking, "When have you experienced a wonderful learning environment? What made it so remarkable? Who was involved and how did they contribute?" will generate a very different response than "What was it like when you were in school?" AI is a highly participatory process that seeks to engage all the stakeholders in the creation of a common vision thereby creating buy-in to potential resulting changes.

Recently, reports of the successful use of AI in health care are beginning to be published. Indiana University incorporated AI into their overall effort to enhance the informal curriculum in their School of Medicine. Participants in their project conducted interviews with medical students to learn about exemplary experiences in professionalism.[42] Members of the faculty at the University of Toronto are using AI to further their efforts in interprofessional education.[43] Researchers in nursing care have employed these techniques in studying pain management, care of psychiatric patients, and care of the elderly.[44-46] At the University of Virginia, AI is being used in quality improvement projects such as improving handoff of care and enhancing team functioning.[26,41] By engaging people at all levels of the traditional hierarchies, AI empowers many members of the health-care team and allows them to share the wisdom of their experience. Not surprisingly, those on the "front lines" often have knowledge and insight that can lead to meaningful change when they and the administrative decision makers join in the conversation.

Stories of Transformation using an Appreciative Inquiry Approach

Transformative experiences can occur at any level. When people are encouraged to "notice" the positive and build on it, the process can transform individual relationships, team functioning, and clinical and organizational outcomes. What follows are a few examples of transformation that have come out of the AI initiative at the University of Virginia.

Our initial experience in using AI was an initiative to reinvigorate our graduate medical education program. In the *discovery* phase, faculty and students interviewed one another about a transformative experience in their teaching or learning. One third-year student told the following story about her pediatrics rotation.

The Girl who Giggled

It was early in my third year during my pediatrics rotation: I had the most adorable little patient. She was a 4-year-old little girl, tiny, even for her age, with big round glasses . . . like the little boy from *Jerry McGuire*. I often saw her sitting alone in her big hospital bed watching TV. She had spent as many nights in a hospital bed as her own bed at home. After multiple abdominal surgeries she required a feeding tube for adequate nutrition.

She had nausea and vomiting that we could not control. Every morning I would walk into her room to examine her. Each day she would stare listlessly at me through her big glasses. No matter what cute voice I tried or how many SpongeBob references I made, she would not talk. She would let me listen to her lungs and belly but didn't respond when I asked her questions. Her parents were very kind. They knew I was trying my best and always encouraged their little child to "cooperate with the nice doctor."

Needless to say, this routine grew tiresome very quickly. It was frustrating that this child refused to talk to me day after day. It was even more frustrating that we could do nothing to help her.

One morning just before rounds I was walking by her room and noticed that the attending physician, a pediatric gastroenterologist, was in the room. I had spoken with him but had never seen him with our patient. I snuck into the room to watch and listen. I was shocked. She was sitting in the bed as always, but she was making eye contact with the doctor, smiling, giggling, talking like you would expect from a 4-year-old. It was the first time I had seen her smile in nearly 2 weeks.

Later that day, I went back to visit her. This time I had a game plan. I tried to follow the example set by the gastroenterologist that morning. I didn't let her shyness get to me. Instead I sat on the end of the bed and talked to her. If she didn't answer, I asked another question. Then I stopped asking her about her condition and instead talked to her about things that would concern a 4-year-old. Instead of examining the feeding tube in her stomach, I give her a big tickle.

Within 2 minutes, she was smiling and talking. I noticed that her parents weren't there, and she told me there wasn't anything good on TV. I spent the next

---

30 minutes sitting with her reading Dr. Seuss books. That day was a turning point. It was still frustrating to take care of her because she had a very difficult medical condition. From that day on, however, I actually looked forward to seeing her every morning.

Transformation can also happen on an organizational level. In another AI project at the UVA we worked with the Department of Psychiatry and the inpatient psychiatric unit to improve the transitions in care for patients being discharged. Nurses recognized that their patients were transitioning to outpatient services and being referred to community resources much more quickly than in the past. With changing health-care reimbursement and limited resources, the trend is for psychiatric patients to be admitted for stabilization and crisis management then to have ongoing therapy in a different environment. The inpatient staff was concerned that these individuals might "fall through the cracks" as a result of challenges coordinating care between the university facility and the community service providers.

With the help of the UVA Center for Appreciative Practice, the inpatient psychiatry staff held a summit and invited representatives of the many local service providers as well as some of their clients. We used an AI approach and a visual metaphor of building bridges. The larger group reflected on times when they felt care transitions had been handled particularly well and the providers had fully met the needs of a patient and his or her family. Together the group envisioned what an ideal treatment plan and care transition would look like and then began to brainstorm ways to make their dream a reality.

Many remarkable outcomes emerged from this event. First, we found that not everyone was aware of the variety of resources already available in the community. When one participant identified a need, another stood up and said, "That's exactly what we do!" and proceeded to tell the others about her organization and how it could integrate with others. Plans were made to create a web network to help the groups better communicate with the goal of eventually making this resource available to clients who might want to access services. Additionally, the various participating agencies agreed on a common format for treatment plans that would promote greater consistency for clients. In the months following the retreats, representatives of one of the more experienced community service agencies came to UVA inpatient psychiatry to help educate staff and implement the plan. UVA staff members joined the board of one agency and began volunteering at others. The posters of bridges used during the retreat were prominently displayed at workstations as a reminder of the new commitment to work together.

Relationships were also formed and strengthened. One client who was part of the process commented on how moved he was to see the commitment and dedication of the professionals in the room. Another participant commented on how nice it was to finally be able to put a face with the voice she had spoken to for more than 12 years. We also received the following story from a registered nurse who participated in the summit.

On the Sunday after the summit, during our silent worship hour in Friends' Meeting, I saw three people, professional consumer advocates, who had been at the summit. Though I have respectful and friendly relationships with them, I—and they—have long been aware of tensions, philosophical and historical, between my location in the mental health system and theirs. Sometimes this awareness has been distracting to me in worship. But on this Sunday I was warmed by their greetings, and felt peace and hope as we sat together. I had a sense in the silence that many of the brambles had been cleared in the path that is between us. After the service we talked in the foyer for half an hour. The conversation was hopeful and planful. We wanted to go to lunch together but had logistical problems. The point is that we didn't want the conversation to end, and, I don't believe it will.

One challenge to the use of AI in health care is that it is a time-intensive process. In our experience, the minimum amount of time required to engage in a 4-D process is 8–12 hours. In an industry that functions 24 hours a day 7 days a week and where patient care must always come first, gathering people for that amount of time is difficult. We have also observed that once the retreat is over, people are energized and enthusiastic about their work but when they return to their daily routine, unless the entire system is changing, many of the same challenges and frustrations arise. For this reason, AI cannot be used in isolation. In order to sustain positivity long enough to achieve some of its benefits, there must also be some simple everyday activities that can be employed by individuals. We call these "appreciative practices."

Appreciative Practices: Strategies for Everyday Use of Positivity in Academic Health Science Centers

Over the past several years, our group has identified a number of appreciative practices. Established AI practitioners have previously identified many of these, but they are foreign to the health-care community. These simple concepts, ideas, and activities are ways that we can help infuse positivity in our environment and ourselves. Appreciative practices are not difficult but they do not come naturally, especially in a culture with such a focus on what can go wrong. Nonetheless, with intention, one can incorporate positivity into a personal leadership style. Then, as described by Fredrickson,[1] this philosophy begins to broaden and build. Examples of appreciative practices include the following.

Start With the Positive

- *Appreciative check-in*: this activity is used to create a positive tone at the beginning of a meeting or gathering. Simply ask the participants if someone would be willing to share the story of something that has gone well over the past 24–48 hours. The request can be tailored toward the focus of the meeting if desired. For example, when meeting with a group of students to debrief a rotation, one could start the meeting by asking for a few to share the highlight of the rotation for them. In addition to changing the mood of the group, this technique can also generate important information.
- *Assumption of positive intent*: this tool can be used by an individual or can be a central belief of a group. Conflicts and misunderstandings are inevitable in any work environment. By assuming that we each fundamentally have positive intent, we can change the course of an interaction. For example, imagine someone returns your manuscript draft and you can't find the original text for all the red ink. One could react by assuming that the reader hated it and could find nothing of value in the article. Alternately, one could be grateful that the reviewer put significant time and energy into helping improve the product.

Moving from Negative to Positive

- *The "Flip"*: a wise old saying suggests, "behind every complaint there is an unfilled wish or desire"; the Flip is a way to discover that wish. Rather than focusing on the activities or behaviors you don't want, consider what you would like to have happen. When met with a complaint, simply ask, "What would you like instead?"

- *Reframing*: reframing is a simple shift in perspective. It is a chance to identify the opportunities in any situation. Transitioning to a new curriculum could be seen as an unnecessary shift that will require the recreation of an entire semester's lectures. Alternately, it could be seen as a way to learn new teaching skills and to excite a new generation of students about the subject matter.

Discovering the Positive

- *The unconditionally positive question*: sometimes an open-ended question will not necessarily get to the desired information. The unconditionally positive question shifts the conversation to times that things have gone well. Questions such as "When have you been a part of a high-functioning interprofessional team?" and "What made the team so successful?" can begin to identify the fundamental aspects of a situation that led to the positive experience.
- *Inquiry rather than judgment*: this approach dovetails beautifully with the assumption of positive intent. Suppose a resident orders a number of tests on a patient for which there isn't a clear indication. Rather than assuming that this shotgun approach is the result of a knowledge deficit and is intended to make sure nothing is missed, the attending could stop and inquire: "I wonder if the resident has gotten new information or if a consultant has suggested these tests."
- *Finding the positive deviant*: "Who is doing this really well in our organization? What can we learn from them?" So often in health care "best practice" has not yet been discovered or defined. If it is defined, the best implementation of that best practice in a specific setting may not yet be discovered. But there are often clever and imaginative people who have found ways to do things really well, within our own communities. As demonstrated by the story of the Sternins and child nutrition in Vietnam, actively identifying the "positive deviants" and learning from them can be the starting point for defining best practice or for designing an implementation process that will work in that setting.

Fostering a Culture of Positivity

- *Gratitude*: how many times have you left a lecture thinking "that was amazing . . . that talk will change how I do things"? Have you had a coworker or colleague provide advice that was incredibly useful? These are opportunities to express genuine gratitude. Telling someone that they have done something that was meaningful to you not only makes them feel good, but according to Seligman's[3] work, will also make you happier.

- *The active positive response*: an active positive response can be used to indicate interest in what someone is telling you. If a student you are mentoring comes to your office to let you know that his case study is being published, there are many ways you could respond. An active positive response might be "That's wonderful! When did you find out? Do you know when it will come out?" By validating his accomplishment and then asking for more detail, this type of response implies that you are genuinely interested and share in his excitement.

- *Positive gossip*: gossip is a powerful social tool. Gossip can strongly influence the success or failure of a new faculty member, a new quality improvement initiative, or a department. Gossip can even influence our clinician–patient relationships. Gossip is almost always negative. We can choose instead to use positive gossip, speaking positively about one another and telling positive stories as a part of the background noise of our community life. Positive gossip can create positive rather than negative expectations of one another and our patients.

- *Cocreating visions*: so often our "visions" are created by individuals far removed from those who are charged with carrying out the vision. Making a commitment to cocreate a vision within an organization pays off in the end when that vision must be realized. It requires discipline to ask, "Is everyone in the room who needs to be?" when a vision is being created. It seems so much easier to create the vision with a small group and then "roll it out." But getting the people in the room to cocreate the vision means that it is more likely to be resonant, realizable, appropriate and energizing.

- *Appreciative Inquiry*: when change is needed, using an AI approach can assure that the process is inclusive, positive, and energizing.

The Culture We Can Create

It is not possible, or desirable, to eliminate all aspects of negativity from our culture. We must continue to critically evaluate our performance and rule out worst-case scenarios. These practices make us better practitioners and better teachers. However, it is important for us to recognize the unintended consequences of these actions as well. We have an opportunity to counter the frequent reinforcement of negativity by intentionally incorporating elements of positivity into our daily activities. Balancing the undesirable impact of negativity requires an active search and cultivation of the positive in our workplace. It is as though in academic health care we are predisposed to negativity, just as the pessimist is predisposed by personality traits to focus on the negative. The pessimist can cultivate optimism by purposeful activities. So can health care. Relatively simple activities like those described above can help broaden our perspective and allow both faculty and learners to be aware of the positive aspects of our environment. Perhaps while we are ruminating over a troubling lab result, we could notice someone making an effort to hold the elevator for us. Or while engaged in a heated conversation over the best course of action for a patient, one could pause to appreciate how passionately each team member cares about this patient's outcome. The research summarized above suggests that it is these small, seemingly inconsequential experiences of positivity that lead to remarkable effects. In the business world, it is now becoming accepted that paying attention to affect is not detrimental or unprofessional. Rather, it is being seen as an important factor in the performance of organizations.[37] It stands to reason that increasing positive affect should be equally if not more important in health care where our primary goal is to enhance well-being.

The "wisdom atmosphere" that psychologist and wisdom researcher John Meacham[47] talks about creating in our centers of learning is one in which "there is a supportive network of interpersonal relations in which doubts, uncertainties and questions can be openly expressed, in which ambiguities and contradictions can be tolerated." This kind of open atmosphere is grounded in positive relationship with others, and is fostered by practices like cultivating curiosity versus judgment, by asking the unconditional positive questions, by assuming positive intent. It is in this positive atmosphere that people are free to question, wonder, and create.

References

1. Fredrickson BL. *Positivity*. New York, NY: Crown Publishing; 2009.
2. Gramling R, Epstein R. Optimism amid serious disease: clinical panacea or ethical conundrum? Comment on "Recovery expectations and long-term prognosis of patients with coronary heart disease". *Arch Intern Med.* 2011; **171**(10): 935–6.

3. Seligman MEP. *Flourish*. New York, NY: The Free Press; 2011.

4. O'Brien CW, Moorey S. Outlook and adaptation in advanced cancer: a systematic review. *Psychooncology*. 2010; **19**(12): 1239–49.

5. Cohen S, Doyle WJ, Turner RB, *et al*. Emotional style and susceptibility to the common cold. *Psychosom Med*. 2003; **65**(4): 652–7.

6. Doyle WJ, Gentile DA, Cohen S. Emotional style, nasal cytokines, and illness expression after experimental rhinovirus exposure. *Brain Behav Immun*. 2006; **20**(2): 175–81.

7. Baumeister RF, Bratslavsky E, Finkenauer C, *et al*. Bad is stronger than good. *Rev Gen Psychol*. 2001; **5**(4): 323–70.

8. Osler W. Address to the students of the Albany Medical College, February 1, 1899. *Albany Med Ann*. 1899; **20**(6): 307–9.

9. Osler W. Aequanimitas. In: Reynolds R, Stone J, editors. *On Doctoring*. New York, NY: Simon & Schuster; 1991. pp. 32–7.

10. Lown BA, Manning CF. The Schwartz Center Rounds: evaluation of an interdisciplinary approach to enhancing patient-centered communication, teamwork, and provider support. *Acad Med*. 2010; **85**(6): 1073–81.

11. Groopman J. *How Doctors Think*. New York, NY: Houghton Mifflin; 2007.

12. Vaish A, Grossman T, Woodward A. Not all emotions are created equal: the negativity bias in social-emotional development. *Psychol Bull*. 2008; **134**(3): 383–403.

13. Haizlip JA, May N, Schorling J, *et al*. The negativity bias, medical education, and the culture of academic medicine: why culture change is hard. *Acad Med*. 2012; **87**(9): 1205–9.

14. Pololi L, Conrad P, Knight S, *et al*. A study of the relational aspects of the culture of academic medicine. *Acad Med*. 2009; **84**(1): 106–14.

15. Spickard A Jr, Gabbe SG, Christensen JF. Midcareer burnout in generalist and specialist physicians. *JAMA*. 2002; **288**(12): 1447–50.

16. Aiken LH, Clarke SP, Sloane DM, *et al*. Hospital nurse staffing and patient mortality, nurse burnout, and job dissatisfaction. *JAMA*. 2002: **288**(16): 1987–93.

17. Goodman M, Schorling JB. A mindfulness course decreases burnout and improves well-being among healthcare providers. *Int J Psychiatry Med*. 2012; **43**(2): 119–28.

18. Samenow CP, Spickard A Jr, Swiggart W, *et al*. Consequence of physician disruptive behavior. *Tenn Med*. 2007; **100**(11): 38–40.

19. Plews-Ogan M, Owens J, May N. *Choosing Wisdom: strategies and inspiration for growing through life-changing difficulties*. West Conshohocken, PA: Templeton Press; 2012.

20. May N, Plews-Ogan M. The role of talking (and keeping silent) in physician coping with medical error: a qualitative study'?. *Patient Educ Couns*. 2012; **88**(3): 449–54.

21. Pololi L, Kern DE, Carr P, *et al*. The culture of academic medicine: faculty perceptions of the lack of alignment between individual and institutional values. *J Gen Intern Med*. 2009; **24**(12): 1289–95.

22. Hampton T. Experts address risk of physician suicide. *JAMA*. 2005; **294**(10): 1189–91.

23. Schernhammer E. Taking their own lives: the high rate of physician suicide. *N Engl J Med*. 2005; **352**(24): 2473–6.

24. Cooperrider DL, Whitney D. *Appreciative Inquiry: a positive revolution in change*. San Francisco, CA: Berrett-Kohler Publishers; 2005.

25. Plews-Ogan M, May N, Schorling JB, *et al*. Feeding the good wolf: Appreciative Inquiry and graduate medical education. *ACGME Bull*. November 2007: 5–8.

26. Haizlip JA, Angle JF, Keefe-Jankowski C, *et al*. Successful adaptation of appreciative inquiry for academic medicine. *AI Practitioner*. 2010; **12**(3): 44–9.

27. Seligman MEP, Steen TA, Park N, *et al.* Positive psychology progress: empirical validation of interventions. *Am Psychol.* 2005; **60**(5): 410–21.

28. Plews-Ogan M, Owens JE, May NB. Wisdom through adversity: learning and growing in the wake of an error. *Patient Educ Couns.* 2013; **91**(2): 236–42.

29. McCrae RR, Costa PT Jr. *NEO Inventories: professional manual.* Lutz, FL: Psychological Assessment Resources; 2010.

30. Plews-Ogan M, May N. Wisdom in medicine: the path through adversity [oral abstract presentation]. International Conference on Communication in Health Care, Chicago, IL; October 18, 2011.

31. Isen AM, Rosenzweig AS, Young MJ. The influence of positive affect on clinical problem solving. *Med Decis Making.* 1991; **11**(3): 221–7.

32. Estrada CA, Isen AM, Young MJ. Positive affect facilitates integration of information and decreases anchoring in reasoning among physicians. *Organ Behav Hum Decis Process.* 1997; **72**(1): 117–35.

33. Ashby FG, Isen AM, Turken AU. A neuropsychological theory of positive affect and its influence on cognition. *Psychol Rev.* 1999; **106**(3): 529–50.

34. Isen AM. An influence of positive affect on decision making in complex situations: theoretical issues with practical implications. *J Consum Psychol.* 2001; **11**(2): 75–85.

35. Isen AM, Reeve J. The influence of positive affect on intrinsic and extrinsic motivation: facilitating enjoyment of play, responsible work behavior, and self-control. *Motiv Emot.* 2005; **29**(4): 297–325.

36. Losada M, Heaphy E. The role of positivity and connectivity in the performance of business teams: a nonlinear dynamics model. *Am Behav Sci.* 2004; **47**(6): 740–65.

37. Sy T, Côté S, Saavedra R. The contagious leader: impact of the leader's mood on the mood of group members, group affective tone, and group processes. *J Appl Psychol.* 2005; **90**(2): 295–305.

38. Singhal A, Buscell P, Lindberg C. *Inviting Everyone: healing healthcare through positive deviance.* Bordentown, NJ: Plexus Press; 2010.

39. Zeitlin M, Ghassemi H, Mansour M. *Positive Deviance in Child Nutrition.* New York, NY: United Nations University Press; 1990.

40. Mackintosh UA, Marsh DR, Schroeder DG. Sustained positive deviant child care practices and their effects on child growth in Viet Nam. *Food Nutr Bull.* 2002; **23**(4 Suppl.): S18–27.

41. Helms AS, Perez TE, Baltz J, *et al.* Use of an appreciative inquiry approach to improve resident sign out in an era of multiple shift changes. *J Gen Intern Med.* 2012; **27**(3): 287–91.

42. Cottingham A, Suchman AL, Litzelman DK, *et al.* Enhancing the informal curriculum of a medical school: a case study in organizational culture change. *J Gen Intern Med.* 2008; **23**(6): 715–22.

43. Dematteo D, Reeves S. A critical examination of the role of appreciative inquiry within an interprofessional education initiative. *J Interprof Care.* 201; **25**(3): 203–8.

44. Kavanagh T, Stevens B, Seers K, *et al.* Process evaluation of appreciative inquiry to translate pain management evidence into pediatric nursing practice. *Implement Sci.* 2010; **5**: 90.

45. Bonham E. Appreciative inquiry in youthful offender psychiatric nursing research. *J Child Adolesc Psychiatr Nurs.* 2011; **24**(2): 122–9.

46. Hirunwat P. Appreciative Inquiry based organization development intervention process on satisfaction and engagement of senior patients and sustainability of Sukavet

Institution: a case study of nursing home. *Revista de Cercetare si Interventie Sociala.* 2011; **33**: 56–71.

47. Meacham J. The loss of wisdom. In: Sternberg R, editor. *Wisdom: its nature, origins and development.* Cambridge: Cambridge University Press; 1990. pp. 181–212.

Complexity

ONE CAPACITY THAT DIFFERENTIATES INTELLIGENCE FROM WISDOM is the capacity to understand and embrace ambiguity and complexity. Wise people avoid oversimplification and black-and-white thinking, and they avoid the mistakes that come from ignoring the ambiguous nature of many situations and underestimating their complexity. In the story that follows, Al Gatmaitan tells of a complex situation in which a critical team was breaking down and falling apart. As a leader he dove into the complexity of the situation rather than approaching with black-and-white thinking. It worked and resulted in one of his strongest teams.

In the ensuing chapter on complexity science we are walked through how an appreciation for complexity can help us see below the surface and work within the ambiguous truth of a situation to find the right course of action, help a team come together, balance competing values, and move a community toward the common good.

A Story: Diving into the Mess

Gene Beyt: An Interview with Al Gatmaitan

Al Gatmaitan has been the chief executive officer of the Indiana University Health Arnett Hospital since 2009. His is a remarkable journey in health-care leadership. His start and ongoing inspiration in health care and health-care leadership was his father's solo general practice in a town of 3000 people in rural Indiana. That was in the 1970s. Al progressed from the "environmental services department" of his father's practice, where he vacuumed, emptied trash, and mowed the lawn at the little house that was the office, to "patient access and registration." There he answered the phone and wrote down appointments in a little scheduling book, and he collected the five or ten or fifteen dollars after the encounter that his father had scribbled on a card to tell Al how much to charge.

This early and formative experience allowed Al to be in the presence of what he would later call a "sanctuary of healing and a very genuine relationship approach to care." Despite his father's language barrier, being Filipino in a very rural Indiana and predominantly white community, after 10 years he was a most beloved physician.

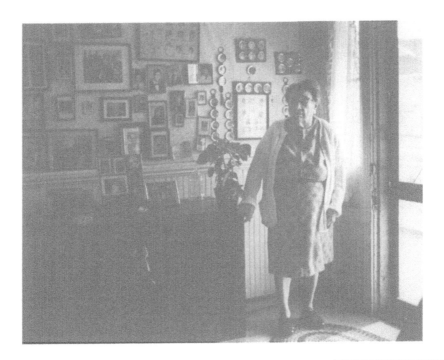

Dr. Gatmaitan achieved this through listening and trying to understand his patients' lives and how he could help. At his father's suggestion Al entered health care, not as a physician but as an administrator working in hospitals and with physicians.

Al's first couple of jobs were in small towns, where he worked with several physicians who practiced in small town environments like his father's. There, he could see how the care process extended from the office into the hospital and back again. It was very obvious to him that the excellent care emanates from the relationship the physician and other health-care professionals have with patients.

This was true in the very most modest settings like his father's house in a town of 3000 and in towns like Tipton, Indiana, with 12 000 people in the entire surrounding county. Years later, Al was asked to draw on his wisdom and his view of patient-centered care and open and lead a brand new hospital that would be a sanctuary of healing. To him the fundamental truth is no different regardless of the size of the enterprise. He is convinced his role is the same as the institution's role—to encourage positive relationships, to create a physical, social and emotional space that promotes healing and health, and to embody these principles at every level of the organization.

After reflection on his personal leadership journey, Al told the following story.

> I have a story I'd like to share related to the experience of creating an organization from scratch. I was charged with opening a new hospital but also creating new medical staff from the scratch of one employee, which was me, and from a brand new facility that was not totally from scratch because it was under the auspices of the larger health system. There was definitely a shadow effect there and an existing culture. But in that effort I was able to see firsthand each ring of influence. In other words, I hired my immediate team and we discussed our objectives, our method of work and how we would relate to each other. We attempted to identify reinforcing cultural norms, such as rituals and symbols that would reinforce the culture we had. Then I was able to observe how each ring expanded its sphere of influence to their direct reports and then they to the next direct reports, and so forth, until we had a thousand or so folks within the same cultural sphere.
>
> Additionally we had multiple physicians coming from multiple different settings, congregating around the hospital and establishing their practices, and they

each had their own culture. So we formed a surgery department. That surgery department was eventually two or three layers away from the CEO office. It was a department that was very effective in cascading the culture of service, of attention to detail, and of building relationships into effective teams. They put their personal mark on it, and created a highly successful surgery department that attracted other physicians and surgeons to come practice here.

One such physician was an orthopedic surgeon who was attracted to a fresh start in this market, liked the surgery department as it was being organized, and made a commitment to move his entire practice to our location. That's the good news. The worry we had was word on the street from the hospitals he had worked in described him as a bull in a china shop. He was also known to be quite difficult to work with interpersonally. Over the first 6 months, the manager, who was outstanding in creating the culture, had several run-ins with this surgeon, who was, on the surface, being quite demanding about how the work should occur. I stepped in and helped convene a team meeting so that we could speak and to listen to one another. It soon became apparent that the surgeon was using what interpersonal skills he had to do complex work with this newly formed team. He was trying to accelerate their growth into a team, and had difficulty expressing what he thought were critical features for this team's performance. His problem was not intent; his problem was not expertise; his problem was that he was under a great deal of time pressure given his busy practice and couldn't sit down and personally orient everyone over and over again. As a result, he got frustrated, acted out, and at times was creating a threatening work environment. However, over the course of some time and conversations, and constantly reinforcing that we were actually on the same page, he and the manager successfully developed a team that could be his champion and be at his side at all times and quickly discern what he needed, and whether they were performing effectively. He became our biggest surgical champion and is still doing very well, feeling quite comfortable in the environment.

So that is a case in which we could have been at odds had we not all taken the time for deeper reflection about the concept of complexity as applied to the formation of this team. Left unattended, the team would have self-organized to act in a certain way, and in this case it was heading in a self-destructive direction. Given some support and direction, the team was able to thrive.

8

Seeing Wisdom in Complexity

Curt Lindberg, Michele Saysana,
John G. Scott, and Robert Lindberg

My Pneumonia

This is the story of my pneumonia. It started on a summer Sunday night at the end of August. I remember waking up in the middle of the night freezing. I was in a deep sleep and woke up so cold I was shivering. For a moment I thought it was winter and then remembered it was August. How strange I thought.

I woke up that morning feeling like I had been run over and wasn't entirely sure whether I had a fever. I knew I had to go to work since it was Monday morning and who was I going to call to get to work for me on that short notice? I needed to relieve the night hospitalist and round on patients. So I did what many of us do in those situations, I took ibuprofen and went to work. Until the afternoon, I was doing well. Then the chills and fever came back once the ibuprofen wore off. I felt like I had been hit by a truck and must have looked like it too since my colleagues sent me home.

When I got home, I went straight to bed. I don't even remember that night. I think I slept through it all—dinner, my kids, my husband coming home from work. The next day proved to be worse. I couldn't get out of bed, let alone go to work. My husband came home that night and asked me how much liquid I had drunk, how many times had I gone to the bathroom, and if I had taken a shower. No to all three I muttered. My husband is a physician, a pediatric anesthesiologist. He asked me the same questions I ask my little patients and their families to figure out how sick they are. Needless to say he wasn't pleased with my responses. So then began the reminders that night to drink. "Michele," he said, "you know you need to drink. You will feel better if you drink and take a shower." I tried to obey like a good patient.

The next day was much like the previous one. The fevers raged on. I started coughing and felt miserable. I was convinced I only had a virus, and would soon feel better. I was hopeful when the fever abated but would nearly cry when the chills came back. Since I was so ill, my husband came home, started an IV, and gave me some fluids in hopes it would make me better. He thought I needed antibiotics and wanted to just prescribe them for me. I didn't think I needed them. I agreed that if I still felt bad the next day I would call my doctor. I didn't want to be one of those doctors who treated themselves. I was determined that I would do it the "right way" and access medical care like everyone should.

That night was awful. I couldn't sleep. I tried to sleep propped up on two pillows. Every time I lay flat, I felt like I was inhaling fluid. My mind raced with scary thoughts. I couldn't figure out what was going on inside my body. The fevers continued that morning but didn't seem quite as bad. My husband listened to my chest and thought I might have pneumonia. So I called my doctor's office. Since I am healthy, I had only been to the office once for a physical about 18 months ago. I spoke with my physician's nurse who told me my doctor was not in the office so I would have to see the physician assistant. With some hesitation, I said, "I'm a pediatrician, and I would really prefer to see one of the other doctors in the office instead of the PA [physician assistant] if possible, please." She replied, "Michele, that is not how it works in our office. If your doctor is not here, you see her PA or NP [nurse practitioner]. If we have one of the other doctors see you, they won't be able to see their own patients." Now normally if I had been feeling well, I would have pushed. However, I was so tired and felt so bad that I just succumbed and said, "OK, what time do you want me to come?"

At the office

At the office, the nurse took my husband and me back to the room. She asked some basic questions after she took my temperature and checked my blood pressure. I had a fever that morning but by the time I went to the office, my temperature was normal. When the PA walked in the room, I remember thinking how young she looked. I have worked with many nurse practitioners and PAs during my career. My personal experience with NPs for my own health care had been very good. With two of my pregnancies, I saw an NP for some of my appointments and was always happy with my care, so I expected this would be the same type of experience. However, it was very different for many reasons. I am usually a very talkative person, but on this day I did not feel like talking. I just wanted to go home and crawl back in my bed. I was already exhausted yet all I had done was take a shower and come to my appointment. The PA was nice enough. She asked how long I had been sick. "How high was your fever?" I replied it was 101.7 that morning, but I was sure that it had been higher. I just hadn't taken my temperature because I couldn't find the thermometer. I also said I was tired and wasn't sleeping well. She then proceeded to ask yes/no questions rapidly. While I answered, my husband sat quietly next to me. She asked about the usual symptoms—cough? Yes; Runny nose? Yes; Eating? No; Vomiting? No. Then she looked in my ears and throat and listened to my chest and heart. She only listened to a few places on my chest, which did not seem thorough enough to me. After her quick exam, she told me everything sounded good and she thought I just had a virus like everyone else. I was so tired I didn't tell her I had missed 3 days of work. I don't think I have ever missed 3 days of work except after I had my three children. She proceeded to prescribe medications used to treat asthma. As tired as I was, I realized this was odd because I don't have asthma. She explained that I probably would still respond to the medications. This was the point when I realized I did not trust her. As sick as I was, I knew that I would not have prescribed those medications in this setting. I wondered if I was just crazy and a hypochondriac. I was disappointed with the visit. I thought I had pneumonia and needed antibiotics, but then I left the office feeling confused. Maybe I did just have a cold virus like the PA diagnosed. All during the visit, I kept wondering why my husband didn't tell her how sick I was. I couldn't understand why he did not speak up. Why didn't he tell her this was not me? Later I realized why.

As we left the office I remember going to get the prescriptions filled at one of my favorite stores and did not even have the desire to get out of the car.

As the day progressed, I was excited since I didn't have any fever the entire morning and through lunch. I was convinced I was better, and the PA was right. I just had a bad virus and was definitely on the mend. Then I lay down for my usual afternoon nap and woke up shaking with fever. Darn—it was back. I felt awful again. My temperature was over 102.

My husband took matters into his own hands and did what he had wanted to do in the beginning. He called one of our close friends, Mark, an internist. I heard him on the phone asking Mark if he could visit us on his way home from the office. He told him I had missed work and continued to have fever after 4 days. Mark was at our house a few hours later standing in my kitchen listening to my story. He took one look at me and instantly knew how sick I was. I could barely stand and talk to him. Again I just wanted to crawl in bed and go back to sleep. He said he was sure I had pneumococcal pneumonia and needed antibiotics. He brought two kinds of antibiotics—one to give me as a one-time injection and other to take by mouth for 10 days.

A bad reaction

I still remember lying in bed after my husband gave me the injection. I was talking with my kids while finishing some dinner, and then my scalp started to itch. I was about to take a shower and thought that would make the itching go away. As I was standing in the shower, I started to have difficulty swallowing. I asked my son to get my husband. I knew what was going on—I was having a bad allergic reaction to the antibiotic. As a matter of fact, I was having an anaphylactic reaction. I stood in the shower thinking to myself I will not die in this shower with dirty hair. My husband came in the bathroom, looked at me in the shower, and told me get out immediately. I kept on washing my hair. My husband who is the pillar of calm even in dire circumstances actually sounded a little panicked. As I got out of the shower and looked in the mirror, I immediately understood why. My face was one giant hive. It was red. My eyes were swollen as were my lips. My voice was hoarse. My medical brain said, "Oh boy, this is *not* good—this is anaphylaxis." My husband immediately gave me the Albuterol inhaler the PA had prescribed earlier that day, two Benadryl tablets, and told me to lie down. He then asked where our nephew's EpiPen was. As Chan brought the EpiPen into our bedroom, I remember telling him, "You know if you give me that you really are going to have to take me to the ER [emergency room] or call 911." He replied, "I know." He sat at the foot of our bed and just watched me for the next 15 minutes or so. He was his calm self on the outside, but he had a somewhat pensive look. I knew in my heart he was worried. As the time went by, my symptoms subsided. My voice was normal. I could swallow. I still itched, but my lip and eyelids weren't as swollen.

It was at that point that I realized how sick I was and that I could have died—died right in my own house in my own bed at age 38 from pneumonia and anaphylaxis. As I recovered over the next few days and finally went back to work after being home for seven days with fever, I realized many things. First, life is precious. In addition, I am a doctor, but when I am sick, I am a patient just like anyone else. When I am ill, I cannot think and process events like I normally would. I am not able to advocate for myself like I normally can when I am well. I also tried to access medical care like everyone does who is not in the medical field and failed to get the help I needed. Part of this was my own fault because I did not tell the PA how sick I was. As a doctor, I know how much I depend on parents of my patients to tell me how sick their child is. As a pediatrician, parents are the best gauge of how their young child is doing. As adults we usually do not have another person with us like a parent to tell the health care provider how sick we are like parents do. This experience has given me a new perspective in my own practice as a pediatric hospitalist. It was very difficult for me to advocate for myself because I was so ill, and I can only imagine what it must be like for parents with ill children or others seeking health care when they are ill.

As I have had months to reflect on this, I asked my husband what he was thinking that day and why he didn't speak up in the office. I'm sure many people might think he was a very passive person and cannot understand why he did not speak up. My husband is anything but passive. He knew from the moment the PA entered the room and started quickly asking questions and making some assumptions that she did not realize how sick I was. He had an expectation that she would treat me for the pneumonia he was sure I had. When she didn't do this, he knew that I needed more help than she was able to provide. He knew how to get it and did.

Sharing my story

After I had recovered from my pneumonia, I shared my story with some of my colleagues who encouraged me to share this story with the office manager and others. When I contacted the office manager, she was very concerned about how I had tried to see a physician and was not allowed to see one. According to her, the nurse should have asked one of the other physicians if they would see me before she told me I had to see the PA. She assured me she would follow up with my physician, the PA, and the nurse who spoke with me on the phone. She also apologized.

I think back to these days that are really a blur and I am thankful that I am here to tell you this story. My story has a happy ending—I am healthy, in better shape than I was before the pneumonia. I also decided to tell my story hoping to make a change in my health system, to make improvements. In my professional role as a pediatrician in quality and safety, I want to make it better for those to come.

I would be remiss if I did not finish my story for you. About 5 months after I thought my story was over, I was at a conference about professionalism. I felt a tap on my shoulder and heard a familiar voice say, "Hello, Michele." As I turned around, my physician was standing there. She began apologizing for not calling me to follow up. She wanted me to know that because of my story the office had made some changes. They changed the policy regarding sick patients requesting to see another physician if their physician was not in the office. Until that moment, I had not been able to bring myself to make an appointment for my yearly physical. I had contemplated switching practices over the last 5 months; but since I was healthy, I had not made the change. During that conversation, I decided I still wanted to see my physician because she knows and understands me. I told her I needed to make an appointment to have my yearly physical. She replied, "You call when you are ready to come see me, and I will be there to see you."

Complexity Science and the Everyday Aspects of Health Care

As Michele's (one of the coauthors of this chapter) story encompasses so many of the everyday, and important, aspects of health care—an illness, encounters with a primary care practice and clinician, medications, and family involvement—it provides a fitting doorway into an exploration of insights from Complexity Science relevant to twenty-first-century medicine. This exploration will entail a primer on Complexity Science and some improvements it has spurred in health care, complemented by stories from two primary care physicians (also coauthors of this chapter) who have devoted themselves to understanding the implications this young science holds for health care and translating its principles into practice.

The Expansiveness of our Metaphors Determines the Expansiveness of our Reality[1]

Progress in science contributes to advancement in medical wisdom. A recent and important advance with broad relevance to medicine is Complexity Science. This science grew partly out of frustration; namely the inability of Newtonian-based models of science to explain the chaotic nature of phenomena.[2] Discoveries and conversations among scientists across disparate fields—mathematics, physics, biology, neuroscience, economics, and sociology—led to its emergence. Edward Lorenz,[3] a meteorologist at the Massachusetts Institute of Technology, noticed odd behavior in computer-generated forecasts and began to question linear weather system models. Cardiologist Ary Goldberger[4] challenged the use of the terms disease and disorder after demonstrating that health is associated with a certain type of physiologic variability and many serious health conditions with a loss of variability and increase in order. Ilya Prigogine, a Nobel Prize-winning chemist, and Isabelle Stengers[5] noticed sudden, radical changes in states of non-equilibrium chemical systems. The renowned biologist Edward O. Wilson and his research partner Bert Hölldobler[6] showed how a simple set of communications among ants led to very adaptable behavior of colonies, or what they called superorganisms. Norbert Elias,[7] the sociologist, observed,

> the basic tissue resulting from many single plans and action of man can give rise to change and patterns that no individual person has planned or created. From the interdependence of people arises an order *sui generis*, an order more compelling and stronger than the will and reason of the individual people composing it.

The work of these and other scholars showed that complex systems have several properties that defy traditional linear models of cause and effect. These discoveries, attributable to what Stephen Hawking called the science of the twenty-first century,[8] are revolutionizing how we understand systems comprised of multiple interacting and interdependent agents.

Scholars and health-care professionals are exploring the implications of Complexity Science for many dimensions of medicine and health care, such as:

- human physiology[9–11]
- primary care[12–14]
- nursing[15–17]
- quality[18–20]
- health-care management[21–26]
- patient safety[20,27]
- public health.[28,29]

Complex systems are everywhere and at all scales in medicine—bacteria, the brain, human body, families, primary care practices, communities, hospitals, health-care systems. The clinician–patient–spouse triad and interaction patterns in Michele's story also compose a complex system.

Aware of the science and its broad relevance for health care, the Institute of Medicine acknowledged health care organizations and processes as complex systems and drew on Complexity Science principles to frame recommendations for the twenty-first-century US health-care system.[30] Nursing has integrated complexity science into its standards for graduate and undergraduate nursing education.

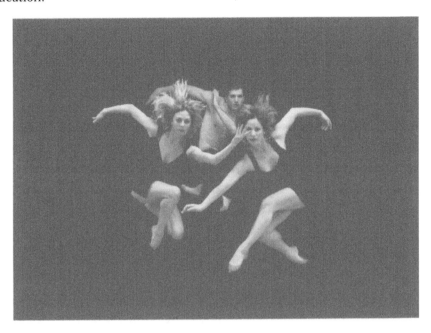

Characteristics and Dynamics of Complex Systems

Complex systems share a number of characteristics and dynamics; self-organization and emergence are two of the most central. Self-organization means that interactions among agents within a system and with other systems spontaneously give rise to order. This ordered state is a consequence of the interactions of the complex system and is not governed by any master controller. Emergence refers to a change in the behavior, state or outcomes in a system that cannot be predicted from the properties of the system's individual agents. In Michele's story, the onset of her disease was an emergent outcome of self-organizing process within her body and an infective agent. The pattern of interaction between the PA, her husband and herself—quick yes/no questions from the PA, short answers from Michele, silence from her husband—was a consequence of their actions and inactions. Since agents in living systems are adaptable, the actions of individual agents influence the behavior of other agents as they are being influenced. Scholars have called this process coevolution.[31]

Resilient, adaptive complex systems are simultaneously ordered and disordered. This condition has been called the edge of chaos and is seen in healthy human physiology.[4] It is also seen in adaptive human interaction. According to both the organizational theorist Ralph Stacey[32] and Ruth Anderson et al.,[33] different perspectives (disorder) are a necessary ingredient for making sense of complex situations and creative problem-solving. Unfortunately, in Michele's story, the PA did not seek the information from Michele's physician/husband. Nor did he offer any.

Complex systems are nonlinear, meaning they may react disproportionately to the size of internal or external perturbations, and that cause and effect are not likely to be proportional. Hence, small changes may ripple through a system and trigger very large changes or large changes may have little effect. This also means behavior of complex systems is inherently unpredictable; surprises may emerge at any time. Sometimes these surprises can be dangerous, like Michele's reaction to the antibiotic injection.

In social systems, Stacey[32] speaks of local interactions generating global patterns; patterns that are paradoxically sustained by ongoing local interactions and, thus, always subject to change. We saw in the interactions between Michele, her husband, and the PA evidence of a pervasive global pattern in health care: an interaction where the professional played the dominant, expert role. She was in charge; she asked the questions. Michele and her husband were complicit in sustaining this pattern, despite their misgivings and despite their experience as physicians. Of course, in this somewhat unusual situation, other factors probably contributed to this pattern. For instance, Michele and her husband may have communicated their lack of trust in the PA. The PA could have been intimidated by encountering two physicians. All of these judgments, actions, inactions, feelings, and assertions of power were part of the brew in what was an encounter lasting but a few minutes. Complex indeed. What is clear is that the dynamics, the pattern of interacting, and the associated power relationships were jointly created and an emergent outcome of a self-organizing process.

Another characteristic of complex systems pertinent to medicine is path dependence. This term suggests that each system's initial conditions, history, and existing patterns of interactions are unique and will affect its future course. It also suggests that the same force acting on seemingly similar systems may stimulate different reactions.[34] The emphasis in traditional science is a search for general findings that apply across similar systems.

Engaging Complexity: Improving Health Care

A growing number of health-care professionals are engaging with these Complexity Science concepts, drawing on them to improve health care and tackle tough problems. Their engagement emanates from some frustration with conventional approaches to quality improvement, change, the patient–clinician relationship, physiologic monitoring, and organizational and team development. New wisdom, new practices, and some encouraging outcomes are emerging as a result. Here are some examples.

- Mortality rates in some neonatal intensive care units are dropping dramatically because of monitoring systems that track changes in the complexity of heart rate variability,[10] an advancement spurred by a growing body of research that demonstrates that changes in physiologic complexity can provide an early warning of the need for life-saving interventions in the critically ill.[35]
- Nursing research has shown that improving connections, the flow of information, and cognitive diversity among staff in nursing homes leads to better resident outcomes;[33] this research is leading to novel interventions aimed at affecting these dynamics.[16]
- Primary care practices that employ complex interventions to improve working interactions among staff are more adaptive, and more capable of achieving the changes needed to become patient-centered medical homes.[14]
- Relationship-centered care concepts[36] and Scott's[37] healing relationships model have been enriched by Ralph Stacey's[32] complex responses process theory.
- As we saw in the last chapter, use of complex improvement processes, like Positive Deviance, are yielding impressive progress on a range of seemingly intractable patient safety challenges like methicillin-resistant *Staphylococcus aureus* (MRSA) infections in hospitals,[20,38] surgical site infections,[39] blood stream infections in dialysis centers,[27,40] and on building cultures of staff engagement.[41]

What follows are two stories of the how Complexity Science has influenced the thinking and practices of two physicians, told respectively by coauthors Robert Lindberg and John Scott.

Story 1: "Good Actions Need the Company of Good Images"[42]

Primary care medicine challenges the most astute clinicians. They must confront myriad confounding variables such as human physiology, psychology, sociology, microbiology, environmental toxins, genetics, and a diversity of cultural practices and beliefs. The business of primary care medicine is equally challenging as it operates on a thin profit margin while attempting to cope with the burden of ever changing regulations from payers and government. Emergencies are never further away than the next phone call, or a door opening into the exam room. The liability exposure is ludicrous, a high wire act that everyone must walk. Practice guidelines that make perfect sense in the policy world rarely live up to their promise in the real world of clinical practice.

I was getting burned out. In my BC world (before exposure to Complexity Science) I was trying to manage a sinking economic ship; a solo practice in primary care medicine. The health-care world was changing under my feet and I was attempting to control and predict the future. This led to an ill-fated dalliance with my local hospital, which took over the administration of my practice for several years. Everyone worked hard to make it successful, but strict adherence to the many rules contained within the hospital employee handbook almost sank my little ship for good. All the good employees left and the patients were frustrated with inflexible management.

Frustration and the Body as a Complicated Machine

As a physician I was uncomfortable with uncertainty both about the future and with those patients with mysterious symptoms. As an expert in diagnostic medicine, I felt obliged to assign causation to all problems but frequently could not. It was frustrating to investigate an ailing patient and not be able to find a broken part, bringing into question my skills or the patient's veracity. I was guided by a concept of the body being a very sophisticated machine with complicated mechanisms, fixable parts and a bewildering array of feedback loops designed to maintain equilibrium. My role as a physician revolved around the following four roles:

1. diagnosing broken parts and seeing they got repaired
2. helping to maintain equilibrium, or homeostasis, by dampening down variations in things such as blood pressure, blood sugar, temperature, hormone levels

3. taking charge of a patient's health, managing and controlling both acute and chronic illness

4. predicting the future so as to take corrective action to avoid problems down the line.

Although always mindful of allowing a patient sufficient time to voice his or her concerns, I also felt compelled to complete a thorough evaluation that involved an "inventory of the parts," both by history and by examination. In my mind there was always a checklist of items to run through, something that every clinician is trained to do. In order to allow enough time for this task I had to seize control of the conversation once I allowed the patient the courtesy of leading off with his or her chief concern. This type of interaction is a form of cross examination, based on the assumptions that I could quickly generate various diagnostic hypotheses and then narrow down the list of possibilities with appropriate discriminating questions and tests. At the end of the interaction I provided the diagnosis and directions for therapy.

This traditional medical interaction is based on some shaky assumptions. The first is that I could quickly inhabit the shoes of my patients, divine their concerns and worries, and understand the import of their words without any ambiguity. The second is that we are the sum of our parts, and optimizing health is a matter of keeping the parts in working order. The third is that I could, with the instruments of modern medicine, be all knowing and all seeing provided I had sufficient information.

Post Exposure to Complexity Science

I disabused myself of these assumptions once I entered the PC phase (post exposure to Complexity Science) of my career. Initially the jargon of Complexity Science was annoying and put me off. However, I came to appreciate the richness of the metaphors and began to see things differently. Science is a way of thinking much more than it is a body of knowledge. One of the achievements of this young science is to suggest a new conceptual framework when assessing the living world. New concepts require a new vocabulary and these words have power if they are productive. A good theory tells you where to look . . . and where not to look. The refreshing aspect of Complexity Science is that it is applicable at all levels of organization within the living world. In other words, the vocabulary provides a common language that can be used by a molecular biologist, a cell biologist, a cardiologist, a pediatrician, and a public health official. At each level there is complex behavior, emergence, and self-organization. Once one grasps the meaning behind these words it changes the way you think about the dynamics of behavior. Now let me inject a word of caution. At each level of organization the rules of behavior are different and shouldn't be confused with one another. Knowing the rules of behavior for a cell provides little assistance for an epidemiologist battling an outbreak of cholera. However, a cell biologist and an epidemiologist both deal with complexity and can utilize the same vocabulary to help them make sense of the problems they confront.

Right around the time I was coming to terms with complexity, the hospital abandoned the administration of my practice. My first step in regaining control of the business of my office was to abandon the hospital's thick employee manual. I had a sense that too many rules imposed rigidity upon an organization. There are many examples from nature of successful living systems organized around simple rules of behavior. As an experiment I decided to start out with three operational suggestions to my staff. The first was we should strive to treat every patient as we would like to be treated ourselves. The second was we had to make more money than we spent each month. The third was there were no other rules. I anticipated I would need to modify this short list as we gained experience but, in point of fact, I have added none since the date they were initiated 10 years ago. The office has no rules for scheduling, appointments, vacation time, lunch breaks, phone etiquette, and so on. If there is any doubt as to what to do we talk it over as we go about our business. No meetings seem to be necessary. A delightful outcome of this strategy has been to dramatically improve the flexibility of the practice. We certainly are more adaptable. The patient population has grown about 30% over this 10-year period, with a resultant increase in income, but I haven't had to hire more staff.

Another gift from Complexity Science has been to shift my focus to the interactions going on among the components of a living system such as the human body, or my hospital network, or my office. The interactions change the components and as the components change they influence subsequent interactions. The interactions within a small office such as mine are chiefly inter-personal and social so I value and nurture these as well as I can. Another type of interaction is with information. An emphasis on facilitating this through early adoption of electronic equipment with flexible software has been critical to the business.

Another insight from Complexity Science, useful to the operational side of my practice, is to fully understand the adage "the only constant is change." The science describes this mathematically. It also illustrates it through examples from nature. The very essence of a living system that survives through time is continual change. In the biologic world the only entity that is static and at equilibrium is dead. So at the start of the day I fully expect the unexpected. Surprise is a given. Variability and change are outcomes of the ongoing interactions within the living world at all levels of organization.

Relationships, Interactions, and Resilience

I don't suggest that anyone else should use as a business strategy my three operational rules of behavior, certainly not a large organization. However, it is an example of gaining some insight from the complexity of the living world and adopting a concept for one's own local use. I emphasize the business of my primary care office first, because as any administrator knows, if the economics don't work you don't have a business. I am not striving to be the next Mayo Clinic. As a matter of fact, I still am comfortable being a solo practitioner. Despite being an endangered species within the health-care world of large networks, my practice is doing well even with having no productivity goals, market analysis, or new income streams. We simply focus on relationships, interactions, flexibility, and resilience and everything else seems to fall into place.

Of course there is another side to a medical practice. Complexity Science has changed the way I look at health and how I interact with patients and how I see my role as a clinician.

Let me give you a few examples.

Complexity Science deals with situations where there are many components interacting with each other on an ongoing basis. It is a very dynamic scenario where nothing remains fixed or static. This scenario is the living world . . . biology, physiology, sociology, politics, management, ecology, to give a few examples. From the standpoint of anatomy, it's helpful to reduce the human organism to a collection of components such as the heart, lung, brain, kidney, and so on; and we have clinicians who specialize on each one of these parts . . . cardiologists, pulmonologists, neurologists, nephrologists. But from a functional standpoint it is more helpful to regard the human organism as a collection of interconnected systems operating at multiples levels, or scales, of organization. A system is a collection of interacting components organized around a common purpose, such as the cardiovascular system, the immune system, the neurologic system. There is a bidirectional flow of information and influence between all the systems so that boundaries are indistinct. There is also a continuous flow of information and energy between all the scales of organization. The molecular level, the cell, the tissue, the organ, the organism, the family, the community are all scales that are simultaneously in play. Clinicians, particularly primary care clinicians, need to embrace this complexity. They need to hold this image in mind when assessing patients and making decisions.

So what are the implications?

First, there are no means to control a complex entity like a living system. You can nudge it perhaps, or influence it, but there is no steering wheel to turn or buttons to push. Efforts to control or direct are, from my perspective, misguided delusions. I need to continually remind myself and my patients of this when we discuss issues such as chronic illnesses or family dynamics. A common marital theme is to wait for the partner to change in order to improve the marriage. "If only my husband would stop drinking" or, "If only she would understand." I call this type of behavior the "Waiting for Godot" syndrome. Two people waiting in vain for some sort of *deus ex machina*. When my daughters were teenagers they taught me a valuable lesson. The only person you can change is yourself. When you change, you will influence people around you.

The second issue concerns assigning causation. "A system is complex when it is sufficiently intricate that the familiar notion of cause and effect is no longer applicable."[11] We humans have a penchant for assigning meaning, plus a cause, to things that happen to us. "Stuff happens" and yes, it happens for a reason. But you can waste a lot of valuable time trying to pinpoint a single explanation. In a complex living system the cause is related to events happening on multiple scales of time and size. A single blood sugar reading in a diabetic is caused by things that are unfolding both on an evolutionary time frame and a microsecond time frame. The blood sugar is also caused by things that are happening within a patient's culture and community but also within the mitochondria of a cell. An unfathomable number of interactions lead to outcomes within a complex system. If you attempt to assign causation you first have to define which scale of time and organization you wish to consider. In diagnosing acute illnesses such as Lyme disease or a heart attack of course you need to know a cause in order to know the treatment. But a lot of medicine deals with chronic illnesses and idiopathic disorders. Here I try not to engage in lengthy discussions with patients or families regarding cause. It can be an empty exercise that takes valuable time away from more pragmatic concerns such as treatment decisions.

For similar reasons, the future is unknowable. We might be able to make a fairly accurate forecast about this afternoon or tomorrow, but not for next month or next year. In our complex world there are just too many variables involved to make accurate predictions about the future. Life emerges unpredictably. At every moment there are many trajectories and many futures that are possible. Just think of all the time we spend trying to predict the weather, or anticipating the direction of stock market indices. Because the underlying dynamics of both these systems are complex, long-term predictions are not possible. It is not because we don't have enough information or the proper computer model. Complexity Science tells us that long-term predictions are impossible because of the inherent uncertainty of complex scenarios. Every day I am asked questions such as these: "My father had heart disease. Do you think I will too?" "Do you think I will get Alzheimer's disease?" "Will my cancer come back?" I try to deflect these questions by pointing out that the future predictions are generally wrong. It is better to concentrate on those things that we can do today that may influence the future favorably for any person that means optimizing their emotional and physical well-being. For an institution it may be positioning the organization so that it can respond to whatever the future brings. Twelve years ago my hospital anticipated that the payment system would shift to capitation and went through an expensive restructuring process as a result. The prediction was wrong. In retrospect a better strategy would have been to become positioned for change rather than making large changes based on a long-term bet.

Finally, the most compelling concept linked with Complexity Science is the idea of emergence. It seems rather magical or mystical. It only occurs where complex dynamics are in play. Most people are familiar with the fact that social insects organized in large colonies, such as ants, bees or termites, can solve almost any problem thrown at them. They have been dominant species for millions of years. The problem-solving capacities of these insects exists only at the scale of the colony. The individual insect has no intelligence. But tens of thousands of ants guided by fairly simple rules of behavior and interacting continuously "scale up" to a form of a superorganism that is very robust and resilient. The wisdom of the colony is an emergent phenomenon that we don't fully understand. Other examples of emergent processes (that we don't fully understand) are consciousness, creative thinking and conversations.

Mysteries to be Solved

There are many instances in primary care medicine where a mystery needs to be solved. In these circumstances I have often found that the traditional medical interview is a hindrance. Familiar to all medical students it is a recipe to be followed so that no relevant information is overlooked. It has its place, but it is a form of interrogation that is one-sided and intimidating. It also assumes that there is only one problem solver in the room.

Inspired by Complexity Science I try to conduct my interviews as conversations, not interrogations, particularly when there is a mystery to solve. By following a simple rule of saying whatever is on the tip of my tongue as soon I enter the exam room, and throughout the interaction, I find a more natural conversation ensues. It has been my experience that as soon as my patients realize that I am following this simple rule, they begin to respond in kind without any coaxing. The result is a surprisingly rich interchange that rapidly cuts to the quick.

In a formal interview (of any type) the agenda is to discuss one topic at a time. The effort to adhere to a predetermined script suppresses the many competing mental images our brain is continuously generating. By contrast, it is much easier to allow ideas to bubble up as they occur. This may lead to a wide range of topics, witticisms and analogies. I find the conversation proceeds more freely because it requires no effort to arrive at whatever is on the tip of your tongue. If one does not censure the expression of these thoughts the comments can be revealing. They also can be embarrassing, surprising, and direct. You may recognize it as a natural form of communication because it is the way children speak.

For example, here is a conversation that I had with one of my patients, TJ, this week.

TJ was struck by a car 5 years ago while riding his bike. He was training for a triathlon. He sustained a spinal cord injury and as a result has paraplegia—paralysis from the waist down. Adjusting to his disability has been a struggle both for him and his family and for me. It is hard to stay ahead of all the emotional and physical consequences that arise from this type of injury. Today he is in for follow-up of abdominal pain that we evaluated at the time of his last visit. The pain was perplexing because he has no feeling below his chest.

TJ: What about those tests we did last week?

Me: Everything checked out fine. That's a new wheelchair, isn't it? Very cool. How is your pain?

TJ: I haven't had it the last 2 days.

Me: You don't look happy about it. Tell me more.

TJ: Um, hard to get out of bed these days. I'm taking my antidepressant but . . .

[Me]: *Often the best response is silence. I wait. Every storyteller needs a listener.*

TJ: Well, you know my son. He's 25 now. He can't seem to get his act together. I worry a lot about him. He's just finishing school now.

Me: I hear you. I have a daughter the same age. We've talked about your son before. I have a hunch there's something more. Is there?

TJ: Sort of.

[Me]: *Storytelling is therapeutic. I wait.*

TJ: My wife. She takes good care of me. All of my nursing needs. I'm lucky that way. But we're not intimate, you know what I mean? Ever since the accident she's cut me off. Not even a hug or a kiss. This wheelchair thing is bad enough. I guess I'm lonely. That's the worst of it.

Me: Do you think she is still angry with you, about the accident?

[I have no idea why I said that. It just came out. He didn't seem to take offense.]

Me: When is it easy for you to get out of bed?

TJ: Lately I have been working as a substitute teacher. I get a kick out of those kids. I never know when I'm going to work, but when I get the call that they need me, it's a good day.

His face lights up in a big smile.

Me: Now I understand where your belly pain is coming from. How can we get you in that school more often?

A creative conversation is analogous to creative thinking. Our brain never stops forming mental images that our minds find attractive or integral to our survival. These images do not occur randomly as they are linked to whatever is engaging our senses or emotions. In a conversation we should allow them full expression because doing so sets off a rapid scanning of numerous interrelated mental images. The churning of these images can lead to helpful metaphors and also creative problem solving.

I have found that a medical conversation that is informal and meandering finds its way to a satisfactory destination with surprising alacrity. Strange as it may seem, taking the indirect route turns out to be more direct.

At the heart of any effective therapy is a healing relationship. When the clinician and patient are guided by the simple rule of saying whatever is on their minds, a relationship is established that is both natural and richly complex at the same time. Moreover by dispensing with the single-minded and directed interview, two humans remain central to a joint discovery process that becomes meaningful to both. Wisdom is an emergent process.

The concepts from Complexity Science are a part of my consciousness now. Here are some of the ways these concepts have changed my role as a physician.

- *Healing begins with a therapeutic relationship*: take advantage of every interaction to deepen that relationship.
- *Focus on enhancing adaptability, flexibility and resiliency*: relinquish delusions of command and control.
- *Be mindful of complexity*: keep in mind that multiple levels of interactions are always in play. Living systems are determined by events that are playing out within time scales ranging from microseconds up to the evolutionary time frame and also within size scales ranging from molecules up to the biosphere. There is no dominant scale of time or size. All are equally important.
- *The most effective communication is through conversations, storytelling and careful listening.*

In reliving Michele's story it is awkward to judge how things could have been different. But when I enter an exam room and see a worried, ill-appearing adult accompanied by a spouse I will typically blurt out something along the lines of "Wow, I see that you are both here. This must be serious! Tell me your story." There is no question that pneumonia can masquerade as a bad upper respiratory virus, or fall closely on the heels of it, so the presumptive initial diagnosis was not unreasonable. However, my own style would have been to have a more free-wheeling conversation so as to allow everyone in that room to give voice to their concerns and expectations. There was a lot of collective wisdom in that room that could have been leveraged into a collaborative decision-making process. Healing is a social phenomenon.

Story 2: Relationships as Powerful Medicine

In 1979, fresh out of family medicine residency, I began practice in a small town in rural Arkansas. I felt well trained, and as a child of the sixties, I was ready to cure disease and change the world. I started out in solo practice, but I always planned to be part of a group; so within a few years I found a like-minded partner. Over the years, we both learned that scientific medical knowledge and medical technology were necessary but not sufficient to take good care of our patients. Our patients had stories to tell us. They were embedded in families and communities and we learned that we ignored those connections at our (and our patients') peril. The stories they told us did not often fit neatly into the diagnostic categories we had learned. We gradually began to realize that the quality of our relationships with our patients had as much to do with how well they did as our diagnostic acumen and the pills we gave them.

One day, for example, a new patient asked me if I would be willing to take on the management of his HIV infection. I was a bit reluctant, since I had only read about HIV/AIDS, and had no experience taking care of patients with HIV infection. I said, "I'll do my best, but I have a lot to learn about this." At the next visit he brought in a large, fat manila envelope full of information about the medical management of HIV infection, and over the next several months taught me his considerable knowledge about the management of AIDS. This relationship stimulated me to learn more on my own, and I eventually became the AIDS doctor for our rural area. Since there were no antiviral agents at that time other than AZT, almost all of these patients, including the first one who was my teacher, eventually died from their disease. In the course of their illnesses, however, I treated many episodes of opportunistic infections and that made the quality of their lives a little better. Our relationships were powerful medicines as well, in both directions. They learned I would not abandon them, and I learned even more about the heroism and courage of men and women living their lives fully in the midst of suffering and death.

My practice partner and I also learned about the business side of medicine. We took turns taking on the job of managing partner. We had a small staff that shared our focus on caring for patients. We were in small office, so there was constant communication among doctors, nurses, and front office staff. Problems were identified early and were solved with input from everyone.

As our practice grew, we took on more partners. Our new partners had different histories, different experiences in practice, different priorities, and different ways of treating patients. These differences created problems in how we cared for patients, but we did not know how to go about team building, and essentially each of us just did our own thing. We hired a larger staff and an office manager, thinking that this would relieve us of the burden of managing the business side of the practice. What it in fact did was isolate us from the front office staff, and create discord and dissent. For example, we had a problem with patients walking in without an appointment. This was frustrating for us and for the front office staff, but the staff felt disempowered to do anything about it. We finally discovered we did not have enough telephone lines to handle the patient appointment calls. The line was always busy, so patients gave up trying to make an appointment and walked in. In our old small office, this problem would have been recognized and solved immediately, but in our new hierarchical system it took months to find and solve it.

Practice was not so much fun anymore, and since I had always been interested in and participated in practice-based research, I left my practice after 21 years and moved to New Jersey to Robert Wood Johnson Medical School to do a fellowship in primary care research, focusing on learning qualitative research methods. It was an exciting time. I was with a group of people from all sorts of disciplines who were doing cutting-edge research in primary care. After the fellowship, I joined the faculty and participated in the design and implementation of a large National Institutes of Health-funded project to help primary care practices improve their care of diabetes, high blood pressure, asthma and hyperlipidemia.[43] This was my first exposure to Complexity Science, since the project was based on the idea that primary care practices were nonlinear complex adaptive systems.

The Complexity of Healing Relationships

Soon after I joined the faculty, I received funding from the Robert Wood Johnson Foundation to pursue my long-term interest in clinician–patient relationships, specifically focusing on how these relationships lead to healing in patients. The project involved long interviews with master clinicians and their patients about their relationships with each other. I had a wonderful time with these interviews. After years of being able to spend only 15 minutes at a time with patients, and no structured time to discuss things with my medical colleagues, I now was able to sit down with both with no time constraints. None of the interviews were shorter than an hour, and one patient interview lasted more than three hours. The doctors and patients told me some amazing stories of healing relationships.

One patient, a practitioner of Christian Science, had been suffering for months with severe congestive heart failure. He described how, when he finally called the doctor, the doctor came to his home, drew his blood, and arranged for his admission to the hospital. Because he had no insurance, rather than calling an ambulance for transport, the doctor brought a wheelchair to the patient's home and took him to the hospital himself.

One doctor said:

> For my panel of patients I am the one that counts. And they count for me, and they know that. And I think there's some aspect of the way that I work where people know that they are known as individuals. They're this person with this vision and this need and care about this. And so there's a sense of who they are and who I am that's alive in the relationship. And I think that's true even with relatively new patients. I think I convey that.

My colleagues and I analyzed hundreds of pages of these interviews and developed a conceptual model of how healing relationships are developed and are maintained.[13] We found there are three essential processes.

1. *Valuing*: that is, master clinicians considered each patient a person of worth, developed a personal connection with each patient, and devoted their full attention (presence) during the interaction.
2. *Appreciating power*: that is, these master clinicians understood that clinician–patient relationships are inherently asymmetrical. They managed this asymmetry by engaging patients as partners in the management of their illness or health, translating medical knowledge so that patients could take charge of their own treatment, and sometimes they used the power differential to push patients to do things they needed to do, but were not quite ready to do on their own.
3. *Abiding*: that is, master clinicians committed themselves to their relationships with patients over time. This involved being accessible for major health events, not abandoning patients even when medical science had little else to offer, and an accumulation of caring actions over time that let patients know that the clinicians cared about them as whole persons.

We realized that this model was scalable; that is, the same processes we saw in clinician–patient healing relationships seemed to be going on in relationships among office staff members in these practices. I saw some practices that were as large as my old practice at the time I left that functioned much better than mine had. I also began to realize that clinician–patient interactions had many of the properties of complex systems at the edge of chaos, and that these healing relationships were emergent patterns of those interactions.

Although I loved research, I discovered that the realities of academic life involved more grant writing than doing research, and that the US National Institutes of Health was not particularly interested in funding research on healing relationships. Also, although I was seeing patients 2 half days a week in a faculty family medicine clinic, I felt like I was not delivering the kind of care I had witnessed in my research. Furthermore, the faculty clinic felt as dysfunctional as the one that I had left in Arkansas. I had learned much from my research about how to take better care of patients, and how practice teams are built, but I was not putting any of that into practice. Fortunately for me, a new opportunity to get reinvolved in patient care came along at just the right time.

A Match Made in Heaven

During the 10 years that I was in New Jersey, I began to develop a connection with a small community in northern Vermont. My wife and I spent vacations there, made friends and eventually bought some property and built a vacation home. As luck would have it, there was a family medicine group owned by the local community hospital that was looking for a family doctor. I moved to Vermont and was able to arrange working for the practice 3 days a week. This schedule allowed me to be accessible enough to my patients to provide the continuity of care I knew they deserved, and it also gave me time to devote to writing and research.

This turned out to be a match made in heaven. Although the practice was larger than the one I left in Arkansas and had an office manager, I experienced none of the dysfunction and isolation that eventually led me to leave my practice in Arkansas. I believe there were several factors that explain this outcome.

The first is history (path dependence in Complexity Science terms). The practice had been founded many years ago by two young family doctors. They intuitively understood healing relationships, and as the practice grew, clinicians and staff were chosen who shared their focus on patient-centered care. When

I arrived the practice already had an established culture that incorporated the processes of healing relationships that I discovered in my research.

The second factor is communication. The practice had regular meetings that involved multiple staff and clinicians. The practice manager had weekly meetings with the front office staff and with the nurses. The clinicians had education meetings every two weeks where clinical topics were presented or cases discussed. There was a monthly meeting of all staff and clinicians. Finally, there was a short quality assurance meeting once a week that was attended by two clinicians and a representative from all the functional areas of the practice: appointments, front desk, nursing, data entry, and transcription. This group identified problems and areas for improvement and worked on solutions for these. All these structured meetings provided the same kind of communication and camaraderie that had happened naturally in my early small practice in Arkansas.

The third factor is stability, which was almost certainly related to the first two factors. The practice had very little turnover in staff or clinicians, so patients felt "known" by almost everyone they encountered in the practice.

The fourth factor is the hospital. Being owned by the hospital allowed us to have infrastructure, including an electronic medical record integrated with the hospital system, that the practice would have had great difficulty acquiring on its own. This did not mean, however, that we were enmeshed in a rigid top-down bureaucracy. The hospital's motto is "We treat you like family," and that statement fits well with the hospital culture. It provides us with the administrative support we need, while at the same time allowing the local culture of the practice to flourish.

The final factor is the state of Vermont itself. Vermont has an ongoing project called "Vermont Blueprint for Health." Our community was one of two pilots in this project. The project funds a community health team based in the hospital and our practice. Our practice therefore has a chronic care coordinator who works with both individuals and the practice's whole population of patients with chronic illnesses. We also have an on-site behavioral health specialist who integrates behavioral and mental health into the care of our patients. Here is an example of how this relational coordination works in the real world.

I walk in to see a new patient, whom we will call Bill Smith. Bill is somewhat disheveled, overweight, and has a flat affect. I manage to get out of him that he wants a "checkup." He tells me that he is disabled and lives with his mother, but he does not know why he is disabled. His blood pressure is 160/100, and his blood sugar is over 200. Later lab work also shows that his low-density lipoprotein is 180. He tells me that he does not take any medicine. I ask for help from the chronic care coordinator and the behavioral health specialist. Working together, they find that Bill has chronic schizophrenia and has consistently refused to take any psychotropic medicines. The chronic care coordinator identifies a sister who agrees to come with Bill to his appointments. The behavioral health specialist finds that Bill is very concrete and will follow instructions to take medicines for his hypertension, diabetes, and hyperlipidemia as long as we give him very specific directions. Bill now comes in for regular appointments with his sister. His blood pressure is 130/80 and his low-density lipoprotein is 80. His diabetes is under better, although not ideal, control—not ideal because he refuses to add insulin to his regimen. He takes his medicines religiously, and also checks his fasting blood sugar regularly, using a glucose meter provided to him by the chronic care coordinator. Without this team approach, Bill would almost certainly have fallen through the cracks in our health-care system and have continued untreated for his serious chronic illnesses.

Lessons from My Medical Journey

What have I learned from my medical journey thus far? I think I can consolidate the lessons into four simple statements. One might be tempted to call these simple rules in the language of complex systems, but my experience and others'[44] suggests that there is nothing simple about human interactions. I would prefer to call these guidelines for interaction among clinicians, patients, colleagues, and staff that make the emergent pattern of healing more likely for patients.

- *History is important*: the history of an individual and the history and culture of an organization determine to a great degree what interaction patterns emerge and how stable and therefore resistant to change they are. Throwing together individuals and systems without an appreciation of the importance of history is almost certain to produce unexpected (and usually unpleasant) consequences. A good example of this is what happened when a multispecialty group that had no history of working with primary care practices acquired my practice in Arkansas. In the first story of what happened when the practice was acquired by the hospital is another good example. Policy makers putting together accountable care organizations in the United States, or similar kinds of collaboratives in other countries, should take notice.

- *Relationships matter*: relationships among patients, clinicians, referral colleagues and staff should be characterized by valuing, appreciating and managing power asymmetries, and abiding.[13] In the words of philosopher Martin Buber, these must be I-Thou rather than I-It relationships—that is, relationships with whole persons rather than collections of symptoms, diseases, job descriptions, or power differentials.[45]
- *Teams work*: clinicians tend to think they care for patients by themselves. My experience is that teams take much better care of both individual patients and populations of patients. Teamwork does not happen by itself, however. As we saw in Chapter 6, a great deal of work has to go into forming the relationships that bond teams into effective patient care units.[46]
- *It takes a village*: Hillary Clinton was referring to education in her book of this name,[47] but engaging the community is as essential for health care as for education. Community can be as broadly or narrowly defined as one wishes, but any useful definition expands community beyond the walls of the practice. In my case, the community turned out to be the whole state of Vermont and its legislature, which provided funding and structure to make community medicine a reality in our practice.

So how does all this connect to Michele's story at the beginning of this chapter? I think her story illustrates how unintended consequences can occur at the level of the individual clinician–patient interaction, the practice, and perhaps the community as well. Everything is always clear in retrospect, so "Monday morning quarterbacking" of this story is neither useful nor relevant. No one in this story, not the patient, the husband, the physician assistant, the receptionist or the doctor wanted or intended a bad outcome to happen, but it did. What I have learned and what my current practice seems to have learned as well is that in complex systems such as primary care practices, unintended consequences are the rule, not the exception. Recognizing this, we find that we must always be mindful of context and outcomes from the level of the clinician–patient interaction all the way to interactions within the community and we must constantly adapt to those changing contexts. Consequently, we never arrive at a perfectly functioning system of care. We can never get there, because there is no "there."

I would argue that clinical wisdom, then, is an emergent pattern of interactions among clinicians, patients, staff, and communities, and that it is constantly cocreated through these interactions.[44] The processes of healing relationships can function at all of these interaction levels, and when present facilitate the emergence of the experience of healing and the growth of wisdom.

References

1. Primack J, Abram N. *The View from the Center of the Universe: discovering our extraordinary place in the cosmos.* New York, NY: Riverhead Books; 2006.
2. Tetenbaum T. Shifting paradigms: from Newton to chaos. *Organ Dyn.* 1998; **26**(4): 21–32.
3. Lorenz E. *The Essence of Chaos.* Seattle: University of Washington Press; 1993.
4. Goldberger A. Fractal variability versus pathologic periodicity: complexity loss and stereotypy in disease. *Perspect Biol Med.* 1997; **40**(4): 543–61.
5. Prigogine I, Stengers I. *Order Out of Chaos: man's new dialogue with nature.* New York, NY: The Free Press; 1984.
6. Hölldobler B, Wilson EO. *The Ants.* Cambridge, MA: Belknap Press; 1990.
7. Elias N. *On Civilization, Power, and Knowledge.* Chicago, IL: University of Chicago Press; 1998.
8. Chui G. "Unified theory" is getting closer, Hawking predicts. *San Jose Mercury News.* January 23, 2000; section A, p. 29.
9. Goldberger A. Nonlinear dynamics for clinicians: chaos theory, fractals, and complexity at the bedside. *Lancet.* 1996; **347**(9011): 1312–14.
10. Moorman R, Waldemar A, Kattwinkel J, *et al.* Mortality reduction by heart rate characteristic monitoring in very low birth weight neonates: a randomized trial. *J Pediatr.* 2011; **159**(6): 900–906.
11. West B. *Where Medicine Went Wrong: rediscovering the path to complexity.* London: World Scientific Publishing; 2006.
12. Crabtree B. Primary care practices are full of surprises. *Health Care Manage Rev.* 2003; **28**(3): 279–83, 289–90.
13. Scott JG, Cohen D, DiCicco-Bloom B, *et al.* Understanding healing relationships in primary care. *Ann Fam Med.* 2008; **6**(4): 315–22.
14. Miller WL, Crabtree BF, Nutting PA, *et al.* Primary care practice development: a relationship-centered approach. *Ann Fam Med.* 2010; **8**(Suppl. 1): S68–79.
15. Anderson R, McDaniel R. Taking complexity science seriously: new research, new methods. In: Lindberg C, Nash S, Lindberg C, editors. *On the Edge: nursing in the age of complexity.* Bordentown, NJ: PlexusPress; 2008. pp. 73–95.
16. Anderson R, Corazzini K, Porter K, *et al.* CONNECT for quality: protocol of a cluster randomized controlled trial to improve fall prevention in nursing homes. *Implement Sci.* 2012; **7**: 11.
17. Lindberg C, Nash S, Lindberg C, editors. *On the Edge: nursing in the age of complexity.* Bordentown: PlexusPress; 2008.
18. Jordon ME, Lanham HJ, Crabtree BF, *et al.* The role of conversation in health care interventions: enabling sensemaking and learning. *Implement Sci.* 2009; **4**(15): 1–13.
19. Lanham H, McDaniel R, Crabtree B, *et al.* How improving practice relationships among clinicians and nonclinicians can improve quality in primary care. *Jt Comm J Qual Patient Saf.* 2009; **35**(9): 457–66.

20. Lindberg C, Norstrand P, Munger M, *et al.* Letting go, gaining control: positive deviance and MRSA prevention. *Clinical Leader.* 2009; **2**(2): 60–7.

21. Begun J, Zimmerman B, Dooley K. Healthcare organizations as complex adaptive systems. In: Mack S, Wyttenbach M, editors. *Advances in Health Care Organization Theory.* San Francisco, CA: Jossey-Bass; 2003. pp. 253–88.

22. Suchman AL. Organizations as machines, organizations as conversations: two core metaphors and their consequences. *Med Care.* 2011; **49**(Suppl.): S43–8.

23. Suchman A, Sluyter D, Williamson P. *Leading Change in Healthcare: transforming organizations using complexity, positive psychology and relationship-centered care.* London: Radcliffe Publishing; 2011.

24. Zimmerman B, Lindberg C, Plsek P. *Edgeware: lessons from complexity for health care leaders.* Irving: VHA; 2001.

25. Lanham HJ, Leykum LK, Taylor BS, *et al.* How complexity science can inform scale-up and spread in health care: understanding the role of self-organization in variation across local context. *Soc Sci Med.* Epub 2012 Jul 4.

26. Lindberg C, Hatch M, Mohl V, *et al.* Embracing uncertainty: complexity inspired innovations at Billings Clinic. In: Sturmberg JP, Martin CM, editors. *Handbook of Systems and Complexity in Health.* New York, NY: Springer; 2013. pp. 697–714.

27. Centers for Disease Control and Prevention (CDC). Reducing bloodstream infections in an outpatient hemodialysis center—New Jersey, 2008–2011. *MMWR Morb Mortal Wkly Rep.* 2012; **61**(10): 169–73.

28. Koopman JS, Longini IM Jr. The ecological effects of individual exposures and nonlinear disease dynamics in populations. *Am J Public Health.* 1994; **84**(5): 336–42.

29. Pearce N, Merletti F. Complexity, simplicity, and epidemiology. *Int J Epidemiol.* 2006; **35**(9): 515–19.

30. Institute of Medicine. *Crossing the Quality Chasm: a new healthcare system for the 21st century.* Washington, DC: The National Academies Press; 2001.

31. McDaniel R, Driebe D. Complexity science and health care management. In: Blair J, Fottler M, Savage G, editors. *Advances in Health Care Management.* Vol 2. Stamford, CN: JAI Press; 1998. pp. 11–36.

32. Stacey R. *Strategic Management and Organisational Dynamics: the challenge of complexity* 6th ed. Harlow: Pearson Education; 2011.

33. Anderson RA, Issel LM, McDaniel RR Jr. Nursing homes as complex adaptive systems: relationship between management practice and resident outcomes. *Nurs Res.* 2003; **52**(1): 12–21.

34. Sterman JD, Wittenberg J. Path dependence, competition, and succession in the dynamics of scientific revolution. *Organ Sci.* 1999; **10**(3): 322–41.

35. Cancio LC, Batchinsky AI, Salinas J, *et al.* Heart-rate complexity for prediction of prehospital lifesaving interventions in trauma patients. *J Trauma.* 2008; **65**(4): 813–19.

36. Suchman AL. A new theoretical foundation for relationship-centered care: complex responsive processes of relating. *J Gen Intern Med.* 2006; **21**(Suppl. 1): S40–4.

37. Scott JG. Complexities of the consultation. In: Sturmberg JP, Martin CM, editors. *Handbook of Systems and Complexity in Health.* New York, NY: Springer; 2013. pp. 257–77.

38. Ellingson K, Muder R, Jain R, *et al.* Sustained reduction in the clinical incidence of methicillin-resistant *Staphylococcus aureus* colonization or infection associated with a multifaceted infection control intervention. *Infect Control Hosp Epidemiol.* 2011; **32**(1): 1–8.

39. Awad SS, Palacio CH, Subramanian A, *et al.* Implementation of a methicillin-resistant *Staphylococcus aureus* (MRSA) prevention bundle results in decreased MRSA surgical site infections. *Am J Surg.* 2009; **198**(5): 607–10.

40. Lindberg C, Downham G, Buscell P, *et al.* Embracing collaboration: a novel strategy for reducing blood stream infections in outpatient hemodialysis centers. *Am J Infect Control.* 2013; **41**(6): 513–19.

41. Lindberg C, Schneider M. Combating infections at Maine Medical Center: insights into complexity-informed leadership from Positive Deviance. *Leadership.* 2013; **9**(2): 229–53.

42. Damasio A. *The Feeling of What Happens: body and emotion in the making of consciousness.* New York, NY: Harcourt Brace; 2000.

43. Balasubramanian BA, Chase SM, Nutting PA, *et al.* Using Learning Teams for Reflective Adaptation (ULTRA): insights from a team-based change management strategy in primary care. *Ann Fam Med.* 2010; **8**(5): 425–32.

44. Stacey R. *Complex Responsive Processes in Organizations: learning and knowledge creation.* New York, NY: Routledge; 2001.

45. Scott JG, Scott RG, Miller WL, *et al.* Healing relationships and the existential philosophy of Martin Buber. *Philos Ethics Humanit Med.* 2009; **4**: 11.

46. Gittell J. *High Performance Healthcare: using the power of relationships to achieve quality, efficiency and resilience.* New York, NY: McGraw Hill; 2009.

47. Clinton H. *It Takes a Village: and other lessons children teach us.* New York, NY: Simon & Schuster; 2006.

Part 3

Leading Wisely

IN THIS FINAL SECTION, A NURSING LEADER AND A PHYSICIAN LEADER reflect on the path of leadership. Angela McBride, former dean of the Indiana University School of Nursing, describes a journey toward wisdom, a journey that has developmental stages which culminate in what she terms the "gadfly" stage, harkening back to Socrates' reflection on his role in the learned community in Greece. Wiley Souba describes the "being" of leadership, an inward journey that is not as much about knowing as it is about what is happening within. This ontological approach to leadership suggests that our worldviews and mental maps affect the way that we see the world, and can limit us. With awareness, and in embracing a wisdom that is inherent, wise leaders can "re-language" or "reframe" their leadership challenges, opening up whole new spaces in which either the challenge disappears (because it was created by our way of thinking) or a creative solution is found.

9

Leadership and the Journey Toward Wisdom

Angela Barron McBride

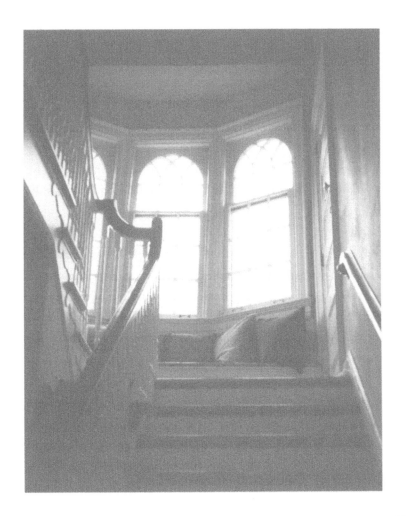

Towards Wisdom

You strive

to develop

yourself. Only to learn

that leaders also must suspend

ego.

You look

for right answers.

Only to realize

that trailblazers ask the spot-on

questions.

You build

your résumé.

Only to discover

that what counts is building hope in

others.

THE CLARION CALL HAS BEEN SOUNDED FOR A NEW KIND OF HEALTH care and new kinds of health professionals. If the twentieth century was characterized by fee-for-service reimbursement, an emphasis on what the physician does, and preoccupation with acute hospital-based care, the twenty-first century is likely to focus much more on bundled-payment models, the value of what intra- and interprofessional teams collectively accomplish (aka outcomes), and care coordination across the health continuum, with an eye to managing chronic health problems so patients stay out of the hospital. The various quality reports produced by the Institute of Medicine in the last dozen years have described the enormous gap between current error-prone realities and desired quality care, noting that all twenty-first-century health professionals must learn to provide patient-centered care as part of interdisciplinary teams, employ evidence-based practices, and utilize quality-improvement methods and informatics solutions.[1-3]

The 2010 Patient Protection and Affordable Care Act (P.L.111-148) calls for the same transformative leadership in the redesign of care because it stresses the achievement of higher quality and greater accessibility at slower-rising costs.[4] The graying of America, which has prompted a renewed emphasis on managing morbidity as a way to manage costs, has further underscored that health is much more than the assessment, diagnosis, and treatment of individual diseases.[5] It must encompass all levels of prevention, rehabilitation, and encouragement of functional ability and quality of life, which can only be accomplished collectively via team-based interprofessional care. The many challenges involved in delivering twenty-first-century health care will not be addressed properly if all health professionals do not practice at the top of their licenses and are not prepared to do their part to lead this change.

Leadership: Beyond Stereotypes

To realize the all-inclusive leadership demanded in the twenty-first century, it is important that certain stereotypes about leadership be dispelled—equating leadership with certain personality traits or with administrative position and associating professional behavior only with what professionals do within the provider–patient relationship. Historically, leadership has often been described in charismatic terms, making it less likely that the more reserved will even think about what form their leadership might take. When leaders are constantly depicted as heroic or rugged individuals—the captain of the ship navigates the shoals; the scientist working alone finds the cure—leadership doesn't seem to be a team sport, which it increasingly must be.[6]

Although most experts would agree that leaders are expected to exhibit some combination of cognitive abilities, emotional intelligence, social capacity, drive, and problem solving, too often the emphasis has been on those characteristics historically identified with men—dominant, forceful, assertive, commanding, formidable, and even tall.[7] This commonplace equation of leadership with being manly certainly gives women a disadvantage in those situations that still seemingly value macho power plays, but they increasingly have documented advantage in settings that place a premium on being perceptive and collaborative, regarded as more feminine traits.[8]

Men might not be quick to describe humility as an important aspect of leadership as one largely female group of leaders did,[9] and the self-effacing socialization that many women have experienced may make it difficult for them to act (or feel) self-confident.[10] Women health-care leaders are expected to be the best, but they may simultaneously be expected not to act self-important, and these warring messages may exert a repressive effect on whether they can unselfconsciously give their all. On the other hand, their male counterparts may have their own difficulty with an emphasis on teamwork, because many have been socialized to take control in a way that may unwittingly silence other voices.

The point is that the gender socialization of the twentieth century can be counterproductive to the team development and collaborative relationships increasingly expected in the twenty-first century. One of the first books to describe male adult development, *The Seasons of A Man's Life*,[11] argued that a man needed a mentor in his twenties and thirties, but was expected to become his own man after the age of 45, the assumption being that he could now manage on his own. Such emphasis on a single hierarchical relationship early in one's career has been questioned, particularly by women, on the grounds that mentors are needed at every career transition; you can learn from a wide variety of helpful collegial and formal relationships and learning must be lifelong.[12]

The health-care professions have traditionally operated from a command-and-control model—physicians "give" orders; others "take" orders—which does not encourage the millions of nonphysicians providing care to speak up about how they see patients and their families through the lens of their particular education/experience. Nurses' roles, for example, are too often limited to those delegated by physicians in a particular setting, so their full potential within the parameters of their licensure is not realized.[13] The invisibility of everything else that nonphysicians do in addition to implementing the medical regimen—for example, surveillance/assessment, patient/family education, counseling, environmental management, and triage—is reinforced when they are largely described as physician extenders. The work of physicians is further exalted if all the other health professions are organized to help them, thus inadvertently increasing the authority gradient.

This authority gradient has proven to be one of the biggest obstacles to the realization of higher quality and safety.[14] Expressing concern, questioning, or even simply clarifying instructions requires considerable determination on the part of team members who may perceive their input as devalued or unwanted. Matters are complicated by the fact that higher-prestige disciplines often think they are more collegial than lower-prestige disciplines perceive them to be. In one study, 42% of nurse leaders said physician disrespect of nurses was common, but only 13% of physicians held that opinion.[15] One possible reason for this difference of opinions is that physicians tend to see good nurses as those who are helpful to them; nurses, on the other hand, want to be appreciated primarily for what they contribute to patient care, not to physicians' effectiveness.[16,17]

The reality is that the various health professions do not know much about each other because they are socialized in separate professional silos, which may only reinforce stereotyped thinking. In an attempt to change that state of affairs, one university had medical students and senior-level baccalaureate nursing students participate in a clinical simulation exercise. In the debriefing, both groups said that they were surprised about what each other knew. When they discussed the shared case, they discovered that each field brought important information to the discussion because they looked at the situation through somewhat different lenses.[18] And that appreciation for the contribution of others is just what is needed for meaningful teamwork in life after graduation.

The differences between and among the health professions is overstated because emphasis is typically placed on what they are able to do when initially licensed or board certified (what competencies are affirmed by this license or certification), rather than on how each health professional changes over the course of a full career. Over time, each health professional who orchestrates a full career is likely to be confronted with the need to assume various functional roles associated with leadership responsibilities—becoming a preceptor, an educator, an administrator, an author, a researcher, a consultant, an officer of a professional association, a fund-raiser, a board member, and/or a policy analyst—and the assumption of these roles presents comparable challenges no matter what the original discipline.

Because the command-and-control model, first associated with monastic life and the military, has historically operated in health-care settings, leadership tended to be equated with administrative position, meaning that even high-status professionals were reluctant to describe themselves as leaders when they did not hold an organizational title. That reluctance operated because the socialization of all health professionals has been primarily to the provider–patient relationship rather than to the systems issues typically identified with administration: How does a physician manage the medical regimen of a complicated patient? How does a nurse organize that complicated patient and her family for discharge? How does a pharmacist prepare a patient on multiple drugs to self-monitor for possible side effects? How does a physical therapist improve the functional ability of a patient with double knee replacements?

This focus on the provider–patient relationship is clinically important, but we now know that the promise of those therapeutic relationships will only be maximized if the context in which care occurs is facilitative of best practices. The physician, nurse, pharmacist, and physical therapist cannot realize their professional best if a culture of safety with appropriate structural supports, information systems, and technological solutions are not in place.[19] That culture of safety will, however, not materialize if only those individuals with administrative titles take responsibility to address those matters, because systems must be clinically relevant and meaningful to all practitioners or otherwise they will not be used. If these systems have no meaning to affected practitioners, they will only work around these practices and those detours will further increase the likelihood of mistakes.

However, if the old views of leadership are dated, what do we put in place so twenty-first-century health professionals can lead the changes being demanded? New views of leadership are needed that apply to all health professionals, and each health profession must prepare its members to exert leadership at every career stage, so we have a workforce prepared to operate at its highest capacity.

Leadership Redefined

Read the leadership literature, and you find that three major views have occupied center stage in the last 8 decades, each new one not supplanting what is in place but further addressing the complexities of being effective in modern times. Early attempts at defining leadership emphasized the qualities all leaders are expected to possess, with "know thyself" being regarded as the key to leadership since Socratic times (*see* Chapter 3 for a discussion of self-reflection as the fundamental capacity for growing in wisdom). But this *leadership as personal* view was eventually criticized because someone can be thoughtful, even charismatic, but fail in achieving institutional mission, values, and goals. Can you be an effective leader if your organization isn't successful in managing its base business? A new view of *leadership as achieving organizational goals* emphasized not just the leader's personality and character but the importance of various instrumental abilities—problem definition and solution, team building, interpersonal and communication effectiveness, resource development (human and otherwise), managing performance, and building the potential of others.

The ability to achieve an institution's long-standing goals was itself ultimately appraised as insufficiently dynamic in a rapidly changing world. Can you be an effective leader if you aren't getting your organization ready for an uncertain future? That is why the literature began to emphasize *leadership as transformational*. In this view, the very meaning of "health," "aging," and "quality of life" keep evolving, so leaders must keep apprised of how the environment keeps changing and develop strategic sensibilities that enable them to find innovative ways of addressing emerging challenges and opportunities.[20] When the fastest-growing demographic group is those aged 85 years and older, it no longer makes sense to treat everyone aged 65 years and older as having the same needs. At a time of constrained resources, business as usual will not work.

To be comprehensive then, twenty-first-century leadership needs to incorporate all three views of leadership in career expectations. In this chapter, leadership is accordingly defined as *inspiring and catalyzing others to realize shared mission and goals in a complex environment that is constantly changing and requiring us to design new ways of achieving our values*. Values do not change with the times, but how they are realized does. The advantage of this definition is that it encompasses the full range of professional behavior from individual performance and productive teamwork to inspiring higher performance in others and creating enduring excellence.[21] It is a definition of leadership that emphasizes teamwork and systems change, not just the masterfulness of any one individual. In order to develop such health leaders, we need to prepare a professional workforce who expect to have full careers, are mentored to exert leadership at each career stage, and who mentor others in each stage.

Leadership at Each Career Stage

It no longer makes sense to focus solely on what health professionals can do once they achieve either their terminal academic degree or their ultimate clinical certification, because that way of thinking ill prepares them for all the challenges that will confront them in a rapidly changing world. The advantage of a career framework, complete with multiple stages, is that no practitioner need start out expecting to be fully developed upon graduation (a comforting thought). Moreover, mentoring—defined as the broad range of developmental relationships whereby more senior individuals work to promote the careers of more junior individuals—comes to play a major role in every transition, and not just in the early period of career development.[22] Like their practice environments, which are constantly changing, thus requiring all organizations to become learning communities so they can adapt to new demands, health professionals must embark on the journey from novice to expert fully committed to lifelong learning, and not just in the sense of accumulating continuing education units to fulfill some regulatory expectation.[23,24]

In this view, a health-care career is a long-term commitment to provide service to others, but one with some expectation of changing for the better in the process (aka growing in wisdom).[25,26] Building on Dalton *et al.*'s[27] classic article on stages of a professional career, Table 9.1 describes five career stages and the mentoring needed at each stage. This developmental framework, like all such others, is primarily meant to be a heuristic device for conceptualizing how the major leadership themes shift over time, pointing the way to the next series of progressive challenges.

TABLE 9.1 Career Stages and Mentoring Needed at Each Stage

Stage	Central Developmental Task	Means	Role of Mentor
Preparation	Assimilating values, knowledge, and clinical/inquiry skills important to a practice profession and health care	Analysis of personal strengths and limitations Formal education Socialization experiences Licensure Certification(s) Membership in professional organizations Strategies for stress management	Model values and practices Encourage problem solving Help set short-term and career goals Guide to experiences that build competencies and expand vision Welcome to profession and identity as fledgling health-care leader
Independent Contributions	Moving from fledgling to competence, while working independently and interdependently with others	Deal with inevitable gap between ideals learned and realities of work setting Ensure that personal practice reflects best practices Demonstrate ability to think, synthesize, and act critically Build teams Develop collegial network Participate in governance Mentor less experienced and less educated	Help navigate inner workings of institution and profession Open doors of opportunity Direct to resources Facilitate networking Keep focus on meeting professional and institutional benchmarks of success Provide feedback so practice, teaching, and/or research improve

Stage	Central Developmental Task	Means	Role of Mentor
Development of Home Setting	Building home setting's image, resources, and infrastructure, while moving personally from competence to expertise	Assume responsibility for programs Engage in strategic planning Head quality improvement efforts Develop junior colleagues Assume major roles in discipline-specific organizations	Help individual learn to juggle multiple projects and responsibilities Provide feedback regarding strategy and tactics Suggest possible "next steps" Help person make best use of others
Development of Field/ Health Care	Shaping future of health care and field/ specialty by exercising power of authority and creating a vision for the future	Consult in area of expertise Serve as advisor to local, regional, national, and/ or international efforts and organizations Set agenda for the future Assume major roles in interprofessional organizations	Provide tips on effective board behavior Recommend for discipline-specific and interprofessional opportunities Sponsor for honors
The Gadfly (Wise Person) Period	Continuing to shape health care and field when no longer constrained by institutional obligations	Coach current generation of leaders Take on special projects that require high-level integrative abilities Speak and write provocatively to challenge new thinking	Help in envisioning post- "retirement" opportunities Recommend for special projects

Note: a version of this table appeared in Chapter 4, Orchestrating a Career, in *The Growth and Development of Nurse Leaders* [20]

In the *Preparation Stage*, the focus is on assimilating the values, knowledge base, and clinical/inquiry skills important to a practice profession and health care. Formal education—undergraduate, graduate, and postgraduate—is important to learn the basics, but socialization experiences (e.g., clinical rotations, internships, residencies, human relations training) are important in applying book learning to real-life situations and developing the qualities at the heart of professionalism. Work as a research assistant, and you soon learn that if things can go wrong in data collection they will go wrong, and problem solving isn't a sometime activity. Take the history of a woman with cardiac problems, and you learn that women can have a heart attack without experiencing the classic male symptom pattern stressed in most textbooks, and understand just how difficult it is for patients to admit to being unwell when they have seemingly vague symptoms.

Achieving licensure is necessary to demonstrate a grasp of fundamentals; specialty knowledge is typically confirmed by certification. It is in this first career stage that one also does certain other groundwork—figuring out personal strengths and limitations; developing the habits of precision (e.g., bookmarking important web sites); learning how to handle stress with emotional equilibrium; deciding which discipline-specific and interprofessional organizations to join. When you are becoming prepared, mentors are important to model values and practices, provide graded challenges that test abilities without overwhelming, teach what is typically not taught in class (e.g., managing time, networking, understanding ethical and proprietary issues), set short-term and career goals, and welcome the individual to the profession as a budding health-care leader. But even in this stage, the individual can mentor others—for example, serving as a big sister or big brother to an incoming student.

In the *Independent Contributions Stage*, the focus is on moving from fledgling to competence while working independently and interdependently with colleagues in the same profession, other health professionals, and a host of technicians and other personnel. Building intra- and interprofessional teams is a task every health professional must face—mentoring the less experienced and less educated; learning how to take advantage of peers who have skills that you do not possess; using those who know more than you do as consultants; developing a sense of collaboration in pursuance of shared goals. At this stage, there is a great deal of tacit knowledge to learn about how to operate within the confines of various organizations.[28,29] Your practice is shaped by the values, history, policies, resources, and mores of the group(s) in which you work and the settings that you frequent. That is why the mentoring that is needed at this stage is largely geared to navigating the inner workings of institutions and professions—opening doors of opportunity, directing to resources, facilitating networking, and keeping the focus on meeting professional and institutional benchmarks of success while understanding how difficult "being new" can be. Even though this is the stage when you are still getting established as a practitioner, it is also a time when you may be asked to be a preceptor for students in their clinical practicums. Coaching them encourages you to have new thoughts about best practices, so there is a reciprocal relationship between helping someone learn something new and getting new insights into the situation.

As practitioners come to realize the extent to which the context of care hinders or supports personal efforts, they are likely to be drawn into governance matters, getting increasingly involved in how the structure can be improved, and that realization frequently propels them to the next career stage. The historic emphasis on independent practice has left many health professionals ill or insufficiently prepared for the systems involvement being demanded these days by the move for hospitals (and all clinical facilities) to become accountable care organizations—integrated delivery systems that align financial incentives, team-based care, electronic health records, and resources to support cost-effective, nonfragmented care—so it has become more important than ever before to help all practitioners become comfortable with and knowledgeable about the systems in which they operate.[30,31]

By the third career stage, *Development of Home Setting*, the individual is learning how to be more of a boundary spanner and how to juggle additional responsibilities and projects. In assuming more responsibility for the development of others and the setting, the practitioner develops further insights into how personal efforts can be supported by the environment, and those perceptions add new depth to his or her understanding of how to move personally from competence to expertise. Where before, the person's focus was on the here and now; now the health professional is increasingly involved in strategic planning for the future, which requires a tolerance for ambiguity and political savvy.

No new vision starts out with a neat 10-point plan, hence the need to learn how you proceed in the face of uncertainty. Knowing what to do is not the same thing as getting what needs doing done, hence the need to be politically astute. Heretofore, the person's focus was on learning the latest and applying that knowledge to care of one's own patients. Now the issue becomes how to get buy-in from others for needed environmental changes when others don't yet understand the need for them or may even be opposed to anything new. Mentors are particularly needed at this stage to provide feedback regarding strategy, particularly how you facilitate junior colleagues who aren't like you, and to help individuals make the best use of others, because most people have some difficulty in using others well when they are used to doing some things themselves, and now have assumed additional responsibilities that call for managerial skills and sensibilities that are still nascent.

By the fourth career stage, *Development of Field/Health Care*, the practitioner takes a more active role beyond the home setting in shaping the profession and health care, doing this by using the authority earned thus far to create a vision for the future. Given success on the home front, the individual is increasingly asked to make larger contributions, serving as an advisor to various organizations and efforts who are interested in achieving similar feats. Any speaking or writing that the person did in the past would have focused exclusively on personal experience, for example, the findings from your research; now that professional is asked to articulate an agenda for the future that requires broader thinking about the specialty for the purpose of setting new directions. As you share your strategic savvy with others, you are forced to analyze anew what you believe, and these reflections often propel your thinking to another level of conceptual complexity. In going elsewhere to consult on what you already know, you will see what that institution is doing and may have new insights into needed next steps at your home institution, thus are better able to mentor your colleagues there who are new to building infrastructure and resources. Even though you are in greater demand as a resource to *other* organizations—serving as a consultant, journal editor, grant reviewer, and/or an officer—you still need mentoring at this career stage. For example, someone who can provide tips on effective board behavior and discuss how you foster generative learning now that you are mentoring relatively senior colleagues.

The fifth career stage, *The Gadfly Period*, is when you continue to shape health care and your discipline but you are no longer employed full time by an institution. While the gadfly is now mainly thought of as a pest, Socrates described the gadfly as one who asks the questions that stir others into life.[32] The gadfly, in this instance, is a truth teller who helps others confront what they might prefer to ignore, but need to tackle for the sake of either the greater good or a deeper meaning. At this stage, when the personal opinions of the professional can no longer be mistaken for the institutional position on this subject, the professional is able to voice views on matters without regard for whether holding an unpopular position will either embarrass the organization or thwart some career ambition. Free of formal organizational obligations, one can be more direct, so the seasoned professional can tackle sensitive subjects more openly than before, and thereby open up an important area for forthright values-based dialogue and more innovative thinking. Former executives can be available for confidential, wide-ranging discussions with the current leadership without having to limit their ideas, as perhaps in the past, to those that can be easily implemented.[33]

In a real sense, the gadfly period is the Wise Person Stage.[34,35] It is not that the individual wasn't impelled by values and professionalism before, but this career stage offers new opportunities to demonstrate compassion and search for meaning. No longer worried about whether you will be invited back to an advisory board, you are freer than ever before to disagree with the majority view. Less personally ambitious, perhaps because you no longer have to prove yourself, the individual can ask whether the right questions have been formulated or the issue is being analyzed with a proper respect for the complexity of the situation. By this career stage, the individual usually has a stronger sense than ever before that the best answers really depend on posing the best questions.[36,37] However, even at this stage, some mentoring is likely to be needed in envisioning post-"retirement" opportunities, because ours is a world that continues to think that professional contributions and having a Medicare card are mutually exclusive categories.

Exerting twenty-first-century leadership presupposes that each health professional is prepared to have a full career, moving over time from promise to momentum to harvest.[38] While some in health care will always choose just to hold a job—good at what they do but what they do doesn't change over time—rather than a career, the high-level practice increasingly required of each professional mandates that normative expectations be shifted in a careerist direction whereby each person is expected to work as a valued team member at the top of her or his license and abilities, and simultaneously prepared to address the systems issues that promote or constrain patient care.

Moving Forward

If health professionals are to exert twenty-first-century leadership, they must operate within interprofessional teams, but interdisciplinary collaboration is still a phrase much discussed without common understandings. Examples of interdisciplinary collaboration have included everything from the blurring of occupational boundaries that occurs in community mental health and when understaffed hospital personnel work together at night, to the establishment of daily nurse–physician planning meetings and combined education and research.[39-41] The Institute of Medicine has asserted that interdisciplinary collaboration is a core competency all health-care professionals need in the twenty-first century, but how to move in that direction remains to be fully described even though there is a call for interdisciplinary research within the National Institutes of Health's

Roadmap and design of Institutional Clinical and Translational Awards to encourage research that spans bench to bed to community.[42]

There remain many stumbling blocks to such collaboration, even though interprofessional education and teamwork is a growing priority of, for example, the Josiah Macy Jr. Foundation.[43] In the twentieth century, thanks to the pervasive influence of the Flexner Report,[44] all of the health professions underwent an extensive process of professionalization, meaning that the various health professions deliberately built their bodies of knowledge, developed practice standards and ethical guidelines, established advance-practice programs, and created certification processes, in order to legitimize their claims to be professional. While these advances facilitated discipline-specific development, they did little to promote cooperation across fields and specialties. Certainly in academia the professions have maintained their distance removed from each other by separate buildings and different school calendars reinforcing the ignorance each discipline has of what the other does.

While there have been repeated attempts to encourage interprofessional practice and education—primary care and geriatric team building in the 1980s and rural initiatives in the 1990s—collaboration tends to disappear when special funding for that purpose evaporates. The time is right to confront health care's Achilles' heel, whereby expertise is present in delivery systems, but inappropriate use of hierarchy and insufficient teamwork prevent the effective sharing of knowledge.[45] The concept of teamwork is resurfacing now with renewed force as important to preventing large numbers of adverse events in expensive acute care, and this time around, chief executive officers and hospital boards are realizing that interprofessional communication affects patient satisfaction, and that affects the bottom line.[46–48]

Collaboration across the health professions is no longer a choice but a necessity, and all concerned need to work on how their prejudices and identities impede or advance care to patients and their families.[49] It has been found that students in the health professions who have been exposed to an interdisciplinary patient safety curriculum come to hold similar values after completing shared instruction even though they started off with substantially different perspectives.[50] There are successful models of interprofessional practice and education in place—some promising ones with an emphasis on the power of coordinated relationships to achieve shared goals (*see* Chapter 6)—and these approaches need to be further tested and then widely disseminated.[51–53]

If mutually respectful interprofessional teams are going to lead the changes we are being asked to set in motion, we need to be much more mindful than we have been to date of whether our language is sufficiently inclusive. The fact that "medicine" regularly gets used as a generic phrase instead of "health care"—complementary *medicine*, *medical* informatics, *medical* center, *medical* record—makes it difficult to tell whether or not the focus of a call for proposals or a practice initiative includes nonphysicians. The same problems associated historically with the confusing generic use of "he" to include "she" hold for "medicine" as an umbrella term.[54] In our language choices, the invisibility of other health team members may be reinforced, making it unclear whether they are even part of a major program. An example of what can happen when there is such lack of clarity is provided by one study of 55 000 clinicians' use of online evidence to support patient care that found the nurses were not sure of their role in initiating information-seeking related to patient care so they were less likely to make use of this resource.[55,56]

This chapter really asks some fundamental questions: Should our focus be to educate for professionalism in medicine or in the health professions as a whole? As each health professional develops the wisdom called for in this volume, is the focus on the development of each profession or on what they can collectively accomplish in confronting the complex issues of our times? What is our primary posture in leadership development and generative learning? These are not trivial questions, because how you look at matters determines to a large extent what you eventually do. Reflection on the part of individuals is useful for self-improvement, but reflection on the part of teams is much more likely to lead to communities of learning prepared to address the thorny issues of the day.

More than a century later, we can applaud what the Flexner Report[44] accomplished in developing each of the health professions. However, the time is ripe now to craft those efforts into a reinvigorated force for collective change, one that focuses on patients, their families, and communities, rather than on discipline-specific self-interest.

References
• • • • • • • • • • • • • • • •

1. Institute of Medicine. *To Err is Human: building a safer health system*. Washington, DC: National Academy Press; 1999.
2. Institute of Medicine. *Crossing the Quality Chasm: a new health system for the 21st century*. Washington, DC: National Academy Press; 2001.
3. Institute of Medicine. *Health Professions Education: a bridge to quality*. Washington, DC: The National Academies Press; 2003.
4. United States Congress. *The Patient Protection and Affordable Care Act* [Act of Congress]. Washington, DC: United States Congress; 2010. Available at: www.gpo.gov/fdsys/pkg/PLAW-111publ148/pdf/PLAW-111publ148.pdf (accessed August 28, 2012).
5. Institute of Medicine. *Retooling for an Aging America: building the health care workforce*. Washington, DC: The National Academies Press; 2008.
6. Northouse PG. *Leadership: theory and practice*. 3rd ed. Thousand Oaks, CA: Sage Publications; 2004.
7. Eagly AH, Johnson BT. Gender and leadership style: a meta-analysis. *Psychol Bull*. 1990; **108**(2): 233–56.
8. Eagly AH. Female leadership advantage and disadvantage: resolving the contradictions. *Psychol Women Q*. 2007; **31**(1): 1–12.
9. Houser BP, Player KN. *Pivotal Moments in Nursing: leaders who changed the path of a profession*. Indianapolis, IN: Sigma Theta Tau International; 2004.
10. Rudman LA. Self-promotion as a risk factor for women: the costs and benefits of counter-stereotypical impression management. *J Pers Soc Psychol*. 1998; **74**(3): 629–45.
11. Levinson DJ. *The Seasons of a Man's Life*. New York, NY: Random House; 1978.
12. Chandler DE, Kram KE. Mentoring and developmental networks in the new career context. In: Gunz H, Peiperl M, editors. *Handbook of Career Studies*. Thousand Oaks, CA: Sage Publications; 2007. pp. 241–67.
13. Bates B. Doctor and nurse: changing roles and relations. *N Engl J Med*. 1970; **283**(3): 129–34.
14. Roberts KH, Madsen P, Desai V, *et al.* A case of the birth and death of a high reliability healthcare organisation. *Qual Saf Health Care*. 2005; **14**(3): 216–20.
15. Cantlupe J. Addressing the disrespect disconnect. *HealthLeaders Media*. March 8, 2012. Available at: www.healthleadersmedia.com/content/PHY-277455/Resolving-the-Disrespect-Disconnect## (accessed August 28, 2012).
16. Prescott PA, Bowen SA. Physician-nurse relationships. *Ann Intern Med*. 1985; **103**(1): 127–33.
17. Back AL, Arnold RM. Dealing with conflict in caring for the seriously ill: "it was just out of the question". *JAMA*. 2005; **293**(11): 1374–81.
18. Reese CE, Jeffries PR, Engum SA. Learning together: using simulations to develop nursing and medical student collaboration. *Nurse Educ Perspect*. 2010; **31**(1): 33–7.
19. Agency for Healthcare Research and Quality (AHRQ). *Patient Safety Primer: safety Culture*. Rockville, MD: AHRQ; 2012. Available at: http://psnet.ahrq.gov/primer.aspx?primerID=5 (accessed August 28, 2012).
20. McBride AB. *The Growth and Development of Nurse Leaders*. New York, NY: Springer; 2011.
21. Collins J. *Good to Great and the Social Sector*. Boulder, CO: Author; 2005.

22. Hargreaves A, Fullan M. Mentoring in the new millennium. *Theory Pract.* 2000; **39**(1): 50–56.
23. Benner P. *From Novice to Expert: excellence and power in clinical nursing practice.* Menlo Park, CA: Addison-Wesley; 1984.
24. Hazer M, Russell S, Fletcher SW, editors. *Continuing Education in the Health Professions: improving healthcare through lifelong learning.* New York, NY: Josiah Macy Jr. Foundation; 2008.
25. Care NS. Career choice. *Ethics.* 1984; **94**(2): 283–302.
26. Pellegrino ED. Professionalism, profession and the virtues of the good physician. *Mt Sinai J Med.* 2002; **69**(6): 378–84.
27. Dalton GW, Thompson PH, Price RL. The four stages of professional careers: a new look at performance by professionals. *Organ Dyn.* 1977; **6**(1): 19–42.
28. Sternberg RJ, Horvath JA, editors. *Tacit Knowledge in Professional Practice: researcher and practitioner perspectives.* Mahwah, NJ: Lawrence Erlbaum; 1999.
29. Eraut M. Non-formal learning and tacit knowledge in professional work. *Br J Educ Psychol.* 2000; **70**(Pt. 1): 113–36.
30. Fisher ES, Shortell SM. Accountable organizations: accountable for what, to whom, and how. *JAMA.* 2010; **304**(15): 1715–18.
31. Shortell SM, Casalino LP, Fisher E. *Implementing Accountable Care Organizations* [policy brief]. Berkeley, CA: Berkeley Center on Health, Economic and Family Security; 2010. Available at: www.mdpso.com/documents/2010_05_Implementing_Accountable_Care_Organizations.pdf (accessed August 28, 2012).
32. Jowett MA, translator. *The Dialogues of Plato.* Vol 1. New York, NY: Random House; 1937.
33. Friel TJ, Duboff RS. The last act of a great CEO. *Harv Bus Rev.* 2009; **87**(1): 82–89, 118.
34. Bateson MC. *Composing a Further Life: the age of active wisdom.* New York, NY: Vintage Books; 2011.
35. Bennis WG. The seven ages of the leader. *Harv Bus Rev.* 2004; **82**(1): 46–53, 112.
36. Riegel KF. Dialectic operations: the final period of cognitive development. *Hum Dev.* 1973; **16**(5): 346–70.
37. Riegel KF. Toward a dialectical theory of development. *Hum Dev.* 1975; **18**: 50–64.
38. Shirey MR. Building an extraordinary career in nursing: promise, momentum, and harvest. *J Contin Educ Nurs.* 2009; **40**(9): 394–400.
39. Mitchell PH, Belza B, Schaad DC, *et al.* Working across the boundaries of health professions disciplines in education, research, and service: the University of Washington experience. *Acad Med.* 2006; **81**(10): 891–6.
40. Baldwin DC Jr. Some historical notes on interdisciplinary and interprofessional education and practice in health care in the USA. 1996. *J Interprof Care.* 2007; **21**(Suppl. 1): S23–37.
41. Clark PC, Dunbar SB, Aycock DM, *et al.* Pros and woes of interdisciplinary collaboration with a national clinical trial. *J Prof Nurs.* 2009; **25**(2): 93–100.
42. National Institutes of Health. *Research teams of the future.* Available at: www.nihroadmap.nih.gov/researchteams/ (accessed August 28, 2012).
43. Josiah Macy Jr. Foundation. *Educating Nurses and Physicians: toward new horizons.* June 16–18, 2010. Available at: www.macyfoundation.org/docs/macy_pubs/JMF_Carnegie_Summary_WebVersion_(3).pdf (accessed August 28, 2012).
44. Flexner A. *Medical Education in the United States and Canada: a report to the Carnegie*

Foundation for the Advancement of Teaching. New York, NY: Carnegie Foundation for the Advancement of Teaching; 1910.

45. Scheele F. The story of health care's Achilles' heel. *Med Teach*. 2011; **33**(7): 578–9.

46. Santana C, Curry LA, Nembhard IM, *et al*. Behaviors of successful interdisciplinary hospital quality improvement teams. *J Hosp Med*. 2011; **6**(9): 501–6.

47. Reeves S, Zwarenstein M, Goldman J, *et al*. Interprofessional education: effects on professional practice and health care outcomes. *Cochrane Database Syst Rev*. 2008; **1**: CD002213.

48. Zwarenstein M, Goldman J, Reeves S. Interprofessional collaboration: effects of practice-based interactions on professional practice and healthcare outcomes. *Cochrane Database Syst Rev*. 2009; **3**: CD000072.

49. Fagin CM. Collaboration between nurses and physicians: no longer a choice. *Acad Med*. 1992; **67**(5): 295–303.

50. Cox KR, Scott SD, Hall LW, *et al*. Uncovering differences among health professions trainees exposed to an interprofessional patient safety curriculum. *Qual Manag Health Care*. 2009; **18**(3): 182–93.

51. Gittell JH, Fairfield KM, Bierbaum B, *et al*. Impact of relational coordination on quality of care, postoperative pain, and functioning, and length of stay: a nine-hospital study of surgical patients. *Med Care*. 2000; **38**(8): 807–19.

52. Hallin K, Henriksson P, Dalén N, *et al*. Effects of interprofessional education on patient perceived quality of care. *Med Teach*. 2011; **33**(1): e22–6.

53. Konrad SC, Browning DM. Relational learning and interprofessional practice: transforming health education for the 21st century. *Work*. 2012; **41**(3): 247–51.

54. McBride AB. Beyond gendered health professions. In: Hager M, editor. *Women and Medicine*. New York, NY: Josiah Macy Jr. Foundation; 2007. pp. 109–45.

55. Gosling AS, Westbrook JI, Spencer R. Nurses' use of online clinical evidence. *J Adv Nurs*. 2004; **47**(2): 201–11.

56. Westbrook JI, Gosling AS, Coiera E. Do clinicians use online evidence to support patient care? A study of 55,000 clinicians. *J Am Med Inform Assoc*. 2004; **11**(2): 113–20.

10

The Phenomenology of Wisdom Leadership

Wiley "Chip" Souba

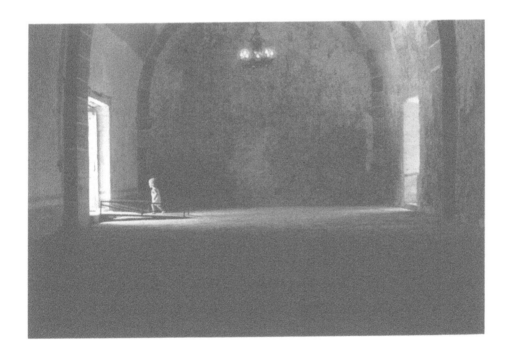

EXCEPTIONAL LEADERSHIP AND WISDOM ARE, NOT SURPRISINGLY, inextricably linked. It would be difficult, if not impossible, to identify an exemplary leader who was not also wise—not so much in the sense of being a "sage"

but in terms of being discerning and exhibiting sound judgment. Willis Harman,[1] former regent of the University of California and president of the Institute of Noetic Sciences, described what we might call "wisdom leadership" to distinguish the type of leadership that is essential for tackling the complex challenges that circumscribe our world today. Nowhere is this need for wisdom leadership greater than in health care.

Knowledge and wisdom are related but different—first, "while knowledge is intrinsically related to action, wisdom is intrinsically related to options; and second, the essence of wisdom is to resolve or integrate divergent problems arising from the nature of human life."[2] We all know individuals who are knowledgeable when it comes to solving problems, but only a handful of these people are truly "wise leaders." They handle the various leadership challenges that crop up in their professional (and personal) lives with grace and ease, without becoming rattled and without shirking responsibility. While we tend to assume that these special leaders possess an unusual gift or specific gene sequence that makes them both wise and unique, what is distinctive about them is that the source of their leadership arises from a unique language. They have mastered a distinctive conversational domain of leadership from which they lead themselves, others, and their organizations. Fortunately, this conversation is available to all of us.

How do we become wise leaders? How do we access wisdom leadership? What is the language of wisdom leadership? These questions are wrestled with in this chapter.

Why Wisdom Leadership and Why Now?

The need for a radical transformation of our health-care system has never been more urgent. Yet, in our hurry to cut costs, our scurry to streamline systems, and our worry about maximizing revenue streams, we tend to forget that we too must change. Some of our most thoughtful scholars have stressed that personal change must precede major systemic (organizational) change (*see* Table 10.1).[3–8]

TABLE 10.1 Individual Change Precedes (Sweeping) Organizational Change

Scholar/Leader	Wisdom Quote
Leo Tolstoy	"In our world everybody thinks of changing humanity, and nobody thinks of changing himself."[3]
George Bernard Shaw	"Progress is impossible without change and those who cannot change their minds cannot change anything."[4]
Peter Senge	"When all is said and done, the only change that will make a difference is the transformation of the human heart."[5]
Jim Kouzes, Barry Posner	"Before you can lead others, you have to lead yourself."[6]
Peter Block	"If there is no transformation inside each of us, all the structural change in the world will have no impact on our institutions."[7]
Victor Frankl	"When we are no longer able to change a situation, we are challenged to change ourselves."[8]

It is becoming increasingly apparent that you cannot lead at your best "out here in the world" unless and until you have a strong leadership foundation "in here." Yet, in our pursuit of technical solutions that require little creativity or collaboration, wisdom may be falling out of favor. Küpers[9] explains:

> Throughout history, wisdom has been seen as a 'supreme' form of human knowledge. . . . [M]ore and more wisdom has become marginalized [and] dominated by technical interests, it has been assimilated and reduced to a psychological construct of cognitive or moral maturation or even as mere exaggerated technical expertise. . . . However, the possession of high levels of knowledge does not in itself mean that a person is wise.

The frenetic pace that characterizes our work lives today leaves little time for quiet reflection and critical thinking (*see* Figure 10.1).

Critical thinking is thinking about your thinking while you're thinking in order to make your thinking better.[10] It requires thinking with discipline and restraint in order to make room—to create an opening—for new linguistic distinctions. Yet, our incessant servitude to the tyranny of the urgent leaves us rushing here and there, often aimlessly, with a latte in one hand and a cell phone in the other. Huizinga[11] warns us of the dangers of information bombardment when he says that there is "something wrong with its assimilation . . .; undigested knowledge hampers judgment and stands in the way of wisdom." General Omar Bradley[12] expressed a similar sentiment when he said: "Ours is a world of nuclear giants

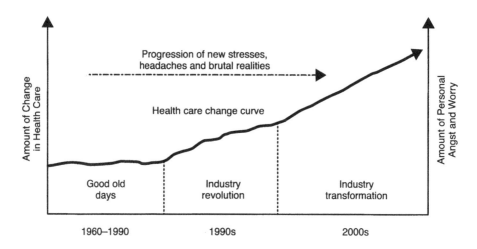

FIGURE 10.1 The amount of gut-wrenching change that pervades our health-care system continues to increase, which contributes to angst, worry, and, at times, despair; wisdom leadership is the portal through which new solutions for our seemingly insurmountable challenges are made available

and ethical infants. If we continue to develop our technology without wisdom or prudence, our servant may prove to be our executioner."

On one level, being frenetically busy makes us feel important. We're constantly in demand, as everybody wants our attention. The expression "to pay attention" has never been more fitting, as we often pay dearly for that which we neglect—our children, our friends, our personal well-being.[13] Merleau-Ponty[14] reminds us that "we are caught up in the world and we do not succeed in extricating ourselves from it in order to achieve consciousness of it." Frenzy and self-reflection rarely go hand in hand.

The inward journey of leadership tends to be neglected for another reason as well—we are inclined to be consumed with looking good, being admired, and measuring up.[15,16] Societal pressures to succeed—and avoid failure—are enormous. Without the capacity to change our taken-for-granted (automatic) ways of being, behaving, and working together in health care, we will default to what is comfortable when we are called to lead and the results we get will be the same—unimpressive, uninspiring, and unacceptable. Schumacher[17] explains:

> The exclusion of wisdom from economics, science, and technology was something which we could perhaps get away with for a little while, as long as we

were relatively unsuccessful; but now that we have become very successful, the problem of [wisdom] moves into the central position.

While knowledge is essential for effective leadership, and arguably more critical than ever, it is not sufficient. "Leaders can be intelligent in various ways and creative in various ways," notes Sternberg,[18] but, "neither trait guarantees wisdom. Indeed, probably relatively few leaders at any level are particularly wise . . .. [This], arguably, is the most important quality a leader can have, but perhaps, also the rarest." Nonaka and Takeuchi[19] clarify:

> Why doesn't knowledge result in wise leadership? The problem, we find, is twofold. Many leaders use knowledge improperly, and most don't cultivate the right kinds. . . . Dependence only on explicit knowledge prevents leaders from coping with change. . . . [Leaders] must also draw on a . . . forgotten kind of knowledge, called practical wisdom. Practical wisdom is tacit knowledge acquired from experience that enables people to make prudent judgments and take actions based on the actual situation, guided by values and morals.

Most of us who work in health care share the conviction that we need more and better leadership. In those moments when we listen intently, that conviction reveals itself as a call for wisdom leadership that comes from deep within. Deep down we want to do something because we are human and we care, but our leadership challenges are daunting and seemingly insurmountable. So we tell ourselves that we are not responsible or that there's nothing much we can do about them. We let ourselves off the hook by saying that they have been around forever. In short, we do not answer the call. This must change.

Wisdom Leadership Lives in Language

When you and I observe someone being a "wise leader" or exercising wisdom leadership, what we see or hear is not a leader or leadership or wisdom per se. What we observe or hear is some way of being, or something said, or some action, which we as onlookers characterize (describe) as wisdom leadership. Moreover, when we witness someone being a wise leader or exercising wisdom leadership, or when we have experienced being led, we observe someone functioning in the sphere of language. More precisely, when you are being a leader and exercising leadership you will be functioning in the sphere of language.

More generally, what is distinctive about human "being" is that the world that shows up (occurs) for us is (in large part) constituted in, shaped by, and accessible through language.[20-23] In other words, access to our life/world is achieved through (granted by) language. Guignon[24] says it this way:

> The prior articulation of the world in language is so all-encompassing that there is no exit from the maze of language. We can never encounter a world as it is in itself, untouched by the constituting activity of linguistic schematizations. . . . On this constitutive view, then, the language in which we find ourselves generates the template through which we come to understand ourselves and the world.

Extrapolating, the way in which our health-care challenges occur for us is shaped by language and is always accessible through language. Said somewhat differently, the way we choose to speak to others and to ourselves about our health-care challenges shapes the way in which those challenges occur for us. To solve our health-care challenges—to exercise wisdom leadership—we need new ways of listening to and talking about these problems (a new conversational domain). New language distinctions open up possibilities for new ways of thinking and new solutions. Language provides actionable access to our way of being and acting in dealing with any leadership challenge.

"We—mankind—are a conversation," wrote Heidegger,[25] by which he meant that conversation is constitutive of human beings. In other words, the way in which the world, others and you yourself occur for you is a function of the conversation that uses you (i.e., your listening). This listening, which includes a set of veiled beliefs, filters, and assumptions "uses" (manipulates) us by providing us a point of view (a context) within which we perceive and interpret reality and orient our actions (Figure 10.2).

Said more generally, the way in which the leadership circumstances you're dealing with occur for you is always shaped by language and always accessible through language.[22,23] And, the way in which the circumstances you're dealing with occur for you will always be matched by (consistent with) your way of being and your actions. If the situation you're dealing with occurs for you as dangerous,

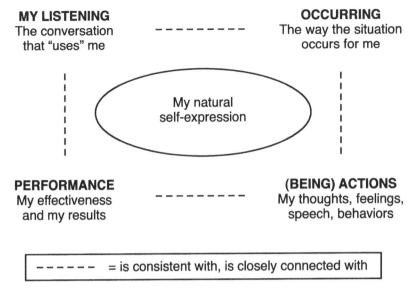

MY LISTENING
The conversation
that "uses" me

– – – – – – – –

OCCURRING
The way the situation
occurs for me

My natural
self-expression

PERFORMANCE
My effectiveness
and my results

– – – – – – – –

(BEING) ACTIONS
My thoughts, feelings,
speech, behaviors

– – – – – – = is consistent with, is closely connected with

FIGURE 10.2 Our effectiveness (performance) as leaders is a function of our listening—this listening, which encompasses a set of veiled beliefs, filters, and assumptions, acts as a context (a point of view) that "uses" (manipulates) us by providing a point of view (a context) within which we perceive and interpret reality and orient our actions; this "listening-occurring" relationship is critical because our way of being and acting always has a profound influence on our effectiveness as leaders—effective leaders use language to recontextualize (reframe, using language) what they are dealing with such that their matched ways of being and actions enhance their leadership effectiveness

you will likely proceed with caution; if it occurs for you as familiar and straight-forward, you will likely proceed with confidence.

This "listening-occurring" relationship is critical because our way of being and acting always has a profound influence on the quality of our lives and our effec-tiveness as leaders. Our effectiveness as leaders, in turn, affects our listening; as we become more empowered the conversations that "use" us become more empowering. Effective leaders use language to recontextualize (reframe) what they are dealing with such that their matched ways of being and actions enhance their leadership effectiveness as their natural self-expression.

Why is a new language of wisdom leadership essential? Because terms like vision, strategy, change, charisma, results, communication, differentiation, character, competence, innovation, and accountability—the words that typically make up the prevailing conversational domain of leadership—provide only limited access to our human ways of being and acting that get in the way of our being wise leaders and exercising wisdom leadership.

Alfred Korzybski,[26–28] a Polish-American engineer and philosopher, maintained that our effectiveness in dealing with the world and its problems is limited by the structure of language. He maintained that human beings do not have access to the objective world; rather, we only have access to our perceptions and to a set of beliefs, which we assume represent direct knowledge of reality. In his masterpiece, *Science and Sanity*,[27] he writes that "all language can be considered as names for unspeakable entities on the objective level, be it things or feelings, or as names of relations."

Korzybski asked: Why do structures built by engineers rarely collapse and, if they do, the basic structural defect can be determined whereas social systems (e.g., health-care systems, economic systems, political systems) routinely collapse (the result being inadequate health insurance, stock market crashes, and insurrections) but the underlying structural defect and requisite solutions are unclear? Korzybski concluded that engineers use a "perfect" language (mathematics) such that the structures they build match the empirical facts and yield anticipated and reliable results. In contrast, when social systems break down it is because

> the structure of the language is not similar to the structure of the situation. When our maps do not fit the territory, when we act as if our inferences are factual knowledge, we prepare ourselves for a world that isn't there.[29]

Just as we need training in how to perform a physical exam on a patient, Korzybski argues we need training in the use of language so we make decisions less by the inferences of our everyday language and more by the actual facts of the circumstances at hand. To solve our complex challenges, he advocated for more deliberate thinking—what we might call wise thinking—in order to make our words more accurately point to the circumstances. A 2005 report from the National Academy of Engineering and the Institute of Medicine[30] underscored the need to identify and apply engineering applications that could improve the delivery of health care. More effective use of the language of engineering in reforming the health-care system should produce structures that match the practical facts and yield better outcomes.

Thought and action are inseparable—they are two sides of the same coin. Prudent action requires prudent thinking. It is through words that we are made human, and it is through words that we are dehumanized.[31] To reform our health-care system, what is needed is a language—a shared conversation—that

> aims not to describe some radically new subject matter which we have
> never yet managed to discuss, but rather to give us the means for ... discus-
> sion of the same one realm of objects to which we have always been trying
> to refer.[32]

Accessing Wisdom Leadership

We can allege, with little debate, that the activity we are calling wisdom lead-ership is a prerequisite for optimal performance both at the individual and organizational level. Leaders need direct access to wisdom leadership, similar to the direct access a researcher has to a database. Current leadership models, however, are based largely on descriptions and explanations (an epistemological model), which provide limited "actionable" access to being an effective leader.[22,23] As Markley and Harman[33] point out, "a science based on description has limits imposed on it by the epistemological limits inherent in the process of descrip-tion." Descriptions alone do not teach what is required to be a leader much as textbooks are not sufficient for becoming a doctor, dancer, or chef. Moreover, in our work, we do not lead from a theoretical approach. To be clear, we lead from the perspective of the way leadership is experienced.

Heidegger[34] challenges the taken-for-granted view of human being as a cogito (an "I") and criticizes the Cartesian predisposition to regard "knowing" as our pri-mary way of interacting with the world. He alleges that "the question of the kind of being which belongs to the knowing subject is left entirely unasked."[34] Arguing that being is primal (we are before we know we are), he argues that "knowing" is a "founded [derivative] mode" of being-in-the-world. In other words, cognition is derivative (a by-product) of some more basic aspect of human existence.

In the prevailing epistemological model of leadership, the source of the leader's performance is taken to be what the leader knows—his or her knowledge, skills, and expertise (Figure 10.3).

The leader is understood as an object with attributes (e.g., know-how, know-what) that informs leadership actions. By contrast, the emerging ontological model of leadership, which maintains that knowing is not enough, is anchored

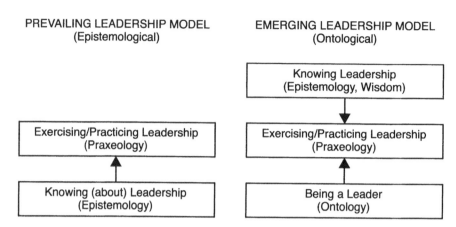

PREVAILING LEADERSHIP MODEL
(Epistemological)

EMERGING LEADERSHIP MODEL
(Ontological)

FIGURE 10.3 Two models of leadership: in the prevailing epistemological model, the source of the leader's performance is taken to be what the leader knows—his or her knowledge, skills, and expertise; by contrast, the emerging ontological model of leadership, which maintains that knowing is not enough, is anchored by the prior nature and primacy of ontology and is based on the premise that it is impossible to act like a leader if one is not being a leader—the source of performance is the leader's way of being and acting (what the leader says and does), which arise in tandem

by the prior nature and primacy of ontology and is based on the premise that it is impossible to act like a leader if one is not being a leader.

Rather than teaching wisdom leadership from a theoretical vantage point, the emerging ontological perspective teaches leadership as it is lived and experienced.[22,23] A distinctive feature of this approach resides in its capacity to disclose our human ways of being and acting that limit our freedom to lead wisely. Ontological leadership maintains that our worldviews and mental maps affect the way we lead and are shaped by and accessible through language—hence, to lead with greater wisdom, mastery of a new conversational domain of leadership is required. Wise leaders "re-language" (reformulate) their leadership challenges so that their naturally correlated ways of being and acting can emerge, resulting in effective leadership. When leaders linguistically unveil limiting contexts, they can create new contexts that shift the way leadership challenges occur for them. The ontological approach to leadership offers a powerful framework for tackling health care's toughest challenges.

In the ontological model, one's performance as a leader is not first and foremost a product of what one knows. Rather, the source of one's performance is largely a function of one's way of being and acting (what the leader says and does), which arise in tandem. As opposed to being perceived as an object with attributes, the leader exists as a clearing that opens up and "discloses" the circumstances and possible realizable futures he or she is dealing with. What one knows (experience, knowledge, expertise) is a combination of both episteme (knowing about) and wisdom (knowing with discernment), which "shed light" on (illuminate) and inform the particular leadership challenge one is confronted with.

How is the inquiry into the meaning of Being to get underway? Heidegger[34] points out that we already have some understanding of Being by virtue of the fact that we are already-always in a world that we are dealing with, which grants us some "pre-ontological understanding of being." The most important feature of human beings, on this account, is that they *care* about their being. We are distinctive among entities in that, for us, our being is *at issue*. To say that our lives are at issue is to say that in our choices and actions at any time we are always taking some stand on what we are, and this stand is crucial to defining our being. To be human is to care about the meaning of our lives and to be concerned about what it is to be. Guignon's[24] elucidation, while erudite and somewhat lengthy, is compelling:

> We are already engaged [in] the attempt to be clear and explicit about our sense of what it means to be.... At the deepest level, truth is envisaged as the emergence of a clearing or opening that releases entities [human beings] from hiddenness [i.e., concealed ways of being that limit our effectiveness].... What we should expect is no longer a final, conclusive answer to the question of Being, but rather a new mode of openness in the asking—a new way of life.... The question of Being ... can be dealt with only by bringing about ... a transformation in our self-understanding of what is at stake in our questioning.

While a mouthful, the essence of the above is highly relevant to the transformation of our health-care system. Much is at stake—incremental change won't cut it as improvements in performance are generally small and offer few, if any, long-term sustainable advantages. What is at stake is the transformation of the Being of human being.

Ways of Being that "Use" and "Create" the Wise Leader

Given the "as-lived" access to leadership provided by the ontological model, we can ask: "What does it mean to be a wise leader who exercises wisdom leadership?" Heidegger[34] understood being as *being-in-the-world*, participating in the world in a process of continuous linguistic "sensemaking" through observing, thinking and feeling in order to make meaning of our relationships with the world. Who we are and who we become, individually and collectively, is constituted in language.

What is my "self"? While I am many things, including an American, a physician, a father, a writer, and so on, none of these is who I am really, for I either did or could exist without being them. While we tend to think of "who I am" as an object with properties, Heidegger[34] argues that human beings are most fundamentally a "clearing"—an opening of conscious intelligibility in which the world shows for us. This clearing both limits and opens up what can "be" (occur) and what can be done. This clearing for action is an "emergent bounded aggregate of ways of being and acting that become possible through language."[35] In other words, this clearing of possibilities doesn't just happen automatically; it "arises out of conversation, so that its [hub and source] is the speech community."[36]

Said somewhat poetically, who I am is the space in which it all shows up. In this space others show up for me, life shows up for me, and I show up for me. It is this space that provides me with access to my way of being and acting in any given situation. How much of the world we will experience is a function of how we understand being and how open we are to it (i.e., what kind of clearing we are).[37] "To exist," says Heidegger, "is essentially . . . to understand."[38] We are not born with this understanding; rather, I acquire the ability to interpret and "take a stand" on my life.[34] Said somewhat differently, how we understand ourselves—as physicians, teachers, scholars, leaders—determines the "shape" of our openness.

Envisaging humans in terms of a space of intelligibility in-the-world is crucial to understanding the ontology of wisdom leadership. While our life-world is generated by neural circuits in our brain, life does not take place in our heads; rather, it happens and is lived out in the clearing that we are. The clearing (context) of conscious intelligibility that I am "governs"[39] the way in which what I'm dealing with occur for me, the way I occur for myself, the way I make sense of my life, and my ways of being, speaking and acting. It is in the clearing that we "be" wisdom leaders. Four ways of being—awareness, integrity, commitment and authenticity—serve as an anchoring foundation (Table 10.2) for being a wise leader and exercising wisdom leadership.[21]

TABLE 10.2 The Being of Wisdom Leadership

Four Ways of Being a Wise Leader	Central Concept
Awareness (being mindful)	Being mindful of the limitations and distortions created by your already-always-listening
Integrity (being your word)	One's word as being whole and complete Keeping your promises; honoring your word when you break them
Commitment (being a stand)	Taking a stand for a future that's bigger than you are, the realization of which fulfills on what you truly care about
Authenticity (being cause in the matter)	A responsible agent (cause in the matter) for dealing with whatever circumstances one is confronted with

Awareness

Awareness, as it is used here, refers to our "voice-over" listening—that is, the background conversation that "uses" us. Early in life, we acquire an involuntary and constant "always-already-listening" that filters and distorts our listening.[23] Once we discriminate this listening as "just there" and on autopilot, it's more like a listening that's thinking for us and manipulating us. Some physicians listen through an already-always-listening of "medicine is no fun anymore." It's the listening (context) they bring to work. They are this listening. Wise leaders are mindful of the limitations and distortions created by their already-always-listening.

Integrity

Integrity—from the Latin word *integritas*—is about one's word being whole and complete.[23,40] "Keeping your word" means doing what you said you would do—that is, keeping your promise. Honoring your word means you don't break it or if you discover you cannot keep your word, you say that you will not be keeping it to those who were counting on your word and clean up any inconvenience or misunderstanding you caused by not keeping your word. Putting integrity into practice as sticking to one's word creates the foundational opportunity for superior performance at both the individual and organizational level. In the absence of this foundation, exceptional performance is not possible and certainly not sustainable.

Commitment

Leaders who are effective are invariably committed to something—a goal, a person, a stand—that is transcendent, big, and bold. Said otherwise, the future you are living into must be a future that's bigger than you are, a future the realization of which fulfills on what is important to you and on what you really care about as a human being. Committing to such a future will give you the power, freedom, and natural self-expression to lead effectively in dealing with the circumstances present in your life right now. Also, it will afford you the necessary direction that allows you to fulfill on what you stand for.

Without standing for a future that's bigger than oneself, the temptation to back off with the smallest derailment will be too great; after all, the future is only a possibility, not a guarantee. Frankl[8] made this very clear when he wrote,

> Success, like happiness, cannot be pursued; it must ensue, and it only does so as the unintended side effect of one's personal dedication to a cause greater than oneself or as the by-product of one's surrender to a person other than oneself.

Authenticity

To lead authentically means to be, regardless of the circumstances of our "thrown situatedness," cause in the matter of our own lives,[34] responsible for creating the clearing that we are. The intriguing term "thrownness" has been used to characterize our inevitable subjection to existence itself.[34] Rather than placing blame or making excuses, authentic leaders take responsibility regardless of the (thrown) mess they find themselves in. Conventionality—"falling prey to the world" or the "they-self"—is the most common form of inauthenticity.[34] Hyde[41] characterizes the authentic leader:

> The authentic self is not one that has managed to escape the everyday thrownness of human being; rather, it is a self that has taken hold of that thrownness "in its own way." It has appropriated the everyday way of being, recognized it, allowed it, and owned it, rather than continuing to be owned by it.

Much of the time we are not as aware of our already-always-listening as we could be, our commitments are self-centered, we are inauthentic, and we do not live as if who we are is our word. Moreover, these disempowering ways of being are often hidden from us. Only human beings can "open up" the world and disclose themselves and their limiting ways of being and, in this sense, "be." Language is the vehicle through which being can be "unconcealed" and understood. This linguistic "disclosure" allows us to unveil our encumbering ways of being and our unproductive behaviors that get in our way of our being effective leaders. Exposing our blind spots and filters, and discerning the limitations they impose on us and our default (automatic) way of being and acting, allow us to create a new context (clearing) such that our behaviors result naturally in our personal best performance for leading in any situation.

Leading Going Forward

The mandate for wisdom leadership has, arguably, never been greater. Cornell historian and political scientist Clinton Rossiter[42] reminds us that we must always keep in mind "both the light and dark sides of human nature—of man's capacity for reason and justice that makes [wisdom leadership] possible, of his capacity for passion and injustice which makes it necessary." Massive and rapid change is needed in health care and we must act soon and wisely. Perhaps our biggest challenge relates to our tendency to fear the unknown and resist change. The reason our health-care challenges seem so daunting and disconcerting may well be not so much their essential complexity as our resistance to letting go of our engrained ways of being and acting. As said eloquently by John Kenneth Galbraith,[43] "Faced with the choice between changing one's mind and proving there's no need to do so, almost everyone gets busy on the proof."

In this chapter we have started to explore a new language (*see* Table 10.3) that gives us improved access to the leadership challenges that confront us in health care. Magalhães[44] tells us that

> the most basic element of organizational action, that is, the basic glue that holds organizations together, is language and languaging.... Language is what allows all action to be coordinated in the organization, and such coordination is achieved by means of organizational members making distinctions about the organization, starting with the first and broadest distinction of them all, which is the concept of "organization" itself.

TABLE 10.3 The Conversational Domain of Ontological Leadership

Term/Phrase
Ontological leadership
Being-in-the-world
Conversation as constitutive of human beings
Cause in the matter
Conversational domain
Committed to a future bigger than you are
The conversation that uses you
Already-always-listening
Linguistic distinction
Clearing
Leadership as-lived
Natural self-expression
Context as a point of view

Said somewhat differently, leadership happens when people construct meaning in action—that is, make sense of what they are doing collectively—in the context of the group's work to accomplish a common purpose or goal.[45]

Wise leaders begin this conversation by clarifying what we value in health care and what kind of health-care system we want to have. Language is the medium leaders use to produce action and get results. But even with the most articulate and clear speech, there is still room for misinterpretation. John Dewey[46] elaborates:

> Experience is already overlaid and saturated with the products of the reflection of past generations and by-gone ages. It is filled with interpretations, classifications, due to sophisticated thought, which have become incorporated into what seems to be fresh naive empirical material. It would take more wisdom than is possessed by the wisest historical scholar to track all of these absorbed borrowings to their original sources.

While Heidegger acknowledged his failure to fully define what it means to be human—"the question of the meaning of Being remains unformulated and unclarified"[34]—his contribution is immense and awakens us to the fact that our lives are embedded in a broader historical project and that we are deeply indebted to our history. To realize this indebtedness is to recognize our burden of responsibility and obligation to the historical context in which we find ourselves.[24]

Effective wisdom practices are initiated by stepping out of our customary ways of experiencing the world, seeing through a different lens, and freeing ourselves from our inherited investments and long-standing, obsolete worldviews. Transforming ourselves and our health-care system begins with dwelling in a different conversation. "It is in and through language that man constitutes himself as a [clearing]"[47] and "it is in and through dialogue that man constitutes himself as a moral agent."[48] All this may sound excessively theoretical, but Peter Russell[49] disagrees:

> It turns out that the wisdom we seek is already there, at the heart of our being. Deep inside, we know right from wrong; this discernment is an intrinsic part of being human. But the quiet voice of this inner knowing is usually obscured by our busy thinking minds, forever trying to help us get the things we believe will bring us peace and happiness and avoid those that will bring pain and suffering. So the real question is: How can we allow the inner light of our innate wisdom to shine through into daily awareness and guide us in our decisions?

As human beings, we can "allow the inner light of our innate wisdom to shine through" because we are those beings for whom our Being is an issue. The construct of that issue is manifested by care.[34] Care, as used here, is not a sentiment. Rather, it refers to being "concerned with [our] ownmost potentiality."[34]

> Because we care about our lives—because who we are matters to us—we have taken some stand on the point of our lives as a whole. . . . In other words, we are always free to make something of our lives as a whole within the confines of the . . . situation into which we are thrown.[24]

Choosing to take this stand is critical because our way of being-in-the-world is the "clearing" in which our leadership concepts and beliefs are shaped; and, the "clearing" that we are defines the contextualizing perspective from which you and I encounter and respond to things in the world.[50]

From whence does this choice to take an authentic stand come from? Heidegger says it derives from transcendence, the primary way—the "basic constitution"—of human "being."[51] This primal way of being is already always there in us but it must be authentically emancipated, a not-so-simple task given our thrownness to inauthenticity. In transcendence, we surpass the "they" and go beyond to our own "for-the-sake-of-which,"[51] the stand each of us takes for making the world a better, healthier place.

References

1. Harman W. *Global Mind Change*. San Francisco, CA: Berrett-Koehler; 1998.
2. Valdesuso C. *Where is the Wisdom We Have Lost in Knowledge?* Brazil: Adizes Institute; 2011. Available at: www.adizes.com/articles/cval-where-wisdom.pdf (accessed December 26, 2012).
3. Tolstoy L. Three methods of reform. In: Tolstoy L. *Pamphlets: translated from the Russian*. Maude A, translator. Ann Arbor: University of Michigan Library; 1900.
4. *George Bernard Shaw: quotes*. Available at: www.whale.to/v/shaw1.html (accessed December 27, 2012).
5. Senge P, Scharmer O, Jaworski J, *et al. Presence: human purpose and the field of the future*. New York, NY: Crown Business; 2008.
6. Kouzes J, Posner B. *The Truth about Leadership*. San Francisco, CA: Jossey-Bass; 2010.
7. Block P. *Stewardship*. San Francisco, CA: Berrett-Koehler; 1996.
8. Frankl V. *Man's Search for Meaning*. New York, NY: Washington Square Press; 1984.
9. Küpers WM. Phenomenology and integral pheno-practice of wisdom in leadership and organization. *Social Epistemology*. 2007; **21**(2): 169–93.
10. Paul R, Elder L. *Critical Thinking*. Upper Saddle River, NJ: Prentice Hall; 2002.
11. Huizinga J. *In the Shadow of Tomorrow*. New York, NY: Norton; 1964.
12. Bradley O. *Quotes by General Omar Nelson Bradley in Wisdom Category*. QuoteWorld; 2012. Available at: www.quoteworld.org/category/wisdom/author/general_omar_nelson_bradley (accessed October 21, 2012).
13. Hallowell E, Ratey J. *Driven to Distraction*. Harpswell, ME: Anchor; 2011.
14. Merleau-Ponty M. *Phenomenology of Perception*. Smith C, translator. New York, NY: Routledge/Kegan Paul; 1962.
15. Souba C. Leading again for the first time. *J Surg Res*. 2009; **157**(2): 139–53.
16. Souba WW. The inward journey of leadership. *J Surg Res*. 2006; **131**(2): 159–67.
17. Schumacher E. *Small is Beautiful: economics as if people mattered*. New York, NY: Perennial; 1975.
18. Sternberg R. *Wisdom, Intelligence, and Creativity Synthesized*. New York, NY: Cambridge University Press; 2003.
19. Nonaka I, Takeuchi H. The big idea: the wise leader. *Harv Bus Rev*. 2011; **89**(5): 58–67.
20. Souba W. The language of leadership. *Acad Med*. 2010; **85**(9): 1609–18.
21. Souba WW. The being of leadership. *Philos Ethics Humanit Med*. 2011; **6**: 5–16.

22. Souba W. A new model of leadership performance in health care. *Acad Med*. 2011; **86**(10): 1241–52.

23. Erhard W, Jensen MC, DiMaggio JJ. *Living with Mastery: what it takes (PDF file of PowerPoint slides)*. May 30, 2011. Harvard Business School NOM Unit Working Paper 11-067; Barbados Group Working Paper No. 11-01. Available at: http://ssrn.com/abstract=1720884 (accessed November 16, 2012).

24. Guignon C. *Heidegger and the Problem of Knowledge*. Indianapolis, IN: Hackett Publishing; 1983.

25. Heidegger M. Holderlin and the essence of poetry. In: Brock W, editor. *Existence and Being*. South Bend, IN: Regnery/Gateway; 1979. pp. 233–69.

26. Korzybski A. *Manhood of Humanity: the science and art of human engineering*. Gloucester: Dodo Press; 2008

27. Korzybski A. *Science and Sanity: an introduction to non-Aristotelian systems and general semantics*. Englewood, NJ: Institute of General Semantics; 1995.

28. Korzybski A. *Alfred Korzybski: collected writings 1920–1950*. Englewood, NJ: Institute of General Semantics; 1990.

29. Weinberg H. *Levels of Knowing and Existence*. Englewood, NJ: Institute of General Semantics; 1991.

30. Reid P, Compton W, Grossman J, *et al.*, editors. *Building a Better Delivery System: a new engineering/health care partnership*. Washington, DC: The National Academies Press; 2005.

31. Montagu A. The language of self-deception. In: Postman N, Weingartner C, Moran T, editors. *Language in America*. New York, NY: Pegasus; 1969. pp 82–95.

32. Stone A. Husserl, Heidegger and Carnap on fixing the sense of philosophical terminology [unpublished]. Available at: http://people.ucsc.edu/~abestone/papers/index.html (accessed January 9, 2013).

33. Markley O, Harman W. *Changing Images of Man*. New York, NY: Pergamon Press; 1982.

34. Heidegger M. *Being and Time*. Macquarrie J, Robinson E, translators. London: SCM Press; 1962.

35. Crevani L. *Clearing for Action: leadership as a relational phenomenon*. Stockholm: KTH Royal Institute of Technology; 2011. Available at: www.diva-portal.org/smash/record.jsf?pid=diva2:414603 (accessed September 17, 2012).

36. Taylor C. *Philosophical Arguments*. Cambridge, MA: Harvard University Press; 1997.

37. Steiner C. The technicity paradigm and scientism in qualitative research. *Qualitative Report*. 2002; **7**(2). Available at: www.nova.edu/ssss/QR/QR7-2/steiner.html (accessed February 13, 2011).

38. Heidegger M. *The Basic Problems of Phenomenology*. Hofstadter A, translator. Bloomington: Indiana University Press; 1982.

39. Heidegger M. *History of the Concept of Time*. Kisiel T, translator. Bloomington: Indiana University Press; 1985.

40. Jensen MC. Integrity: without it nothing works. Interview by Karen Christensen. *Rotman Magazine*. 2009; Fall: 16–20.

41. Hyde RB. Listening authentically: a Heideggerian perspective on interpersonal communication. In: Carter K, Presnell M, editors. *Interpretive Approaches to Interpersonal Communication*. Albany, NY: SUNY Press; 1994. pp 179–95.

42. Rossiter C. Introduction. In: Madison J. *The Federalist Papers*. New York: A Mentor Book; 1961. pp. xiv–xv.

43. Galbraith J. *The Essential Galbraith*. New York, NY: Houghton Mifflin Harcourt; 2001.

44. Magalhães R. *The Organizational Implementation of Information Systems: Towards a New Theory* [dissertation]. London: The London School of Economics and Political Science; 1999. Available at: www.lse.ac.uk/collections/informationSystems/pdf/theses/magalhaes. pdf (accessed May 9, 2010).

45. Drath W. *The Deep Blue Sea*. San Francisco, CA: Jossey-Bass; 2001.

46. Dewey J. *Experience and Nature*. New York, NY: Dover Publications; 1958.

47. Benveniste E. *Subjectivity in Language: problems in general linguistics*. Meek ME, translator. Miami, FL: University of Miami Press; 1971.

48. Braten S. *Intersubjective Communication and Emotion in Early Ontogeny*. New York, NY: Cambridge University Press; 1998.

49. Russell P. *What is Wisdom?* Available at: www.peterrussell.com/SP/Wisdom.php (accessed December 18, 2012).

50. Hyde RB. *Saying the Clearing: a Heideggerian analysis of the ontological rhetoric of Werner Erhard* [dissertation]. Los Angeles: University of Southern California; 1991.

51. Heidegger M. *The Metaphysical Foundations of Logic*. Heim M, translator. Bloomington: Indiana University Press; 1984.

Coda: You Were Made for This

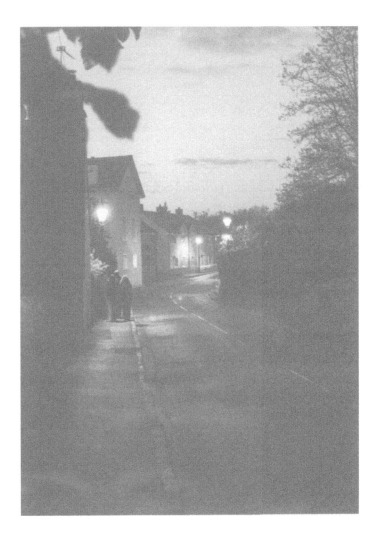

THESE ARE CHALLENGING TIMES IN HEALTH CARE. LEADING CHANGE IN such times is a daunting task. But as healers, *we know about things like compassion, and meaning, and gratitude, and joy.* Wisdom leadership builds on capacities that we each have as human beings, and that we have honed as healers, capacities for deep connection with others, for compassion, for awareness of our own thought processes and limitations, for creating language that communicates our most profound thoughts, for appreciating complexity and for creating meaning in our lives. These capacities lead us to wisdom, to our best selves. By fostering these capacities in our students, residents, faculty, and staff, we as leaders move our Academic Health Science Centers toward wisdom and compassion. This is, in fact, *what we were made for*.

Margaret Plews-Ogan
Gene Beyt
August 2013

You Were Made For This

One of the most calming and powerful actions you can do
To intervene in a stormy world
Is to stand up and show your soul.
Soul on deck shines like gold in dark times.
The light of the soul throws sparks, can send up flares,
Builds signal fires, causes proper matters to catch fire.
To display the lantern or soul in shadowy dark times like these,
To be fierce and to show mercy toward others;
Both are acts of immense bravery and greatest necessity.
Struggling souls catch light from other souls who are fully lit and willing to
   show it.

—Clarissa Pinkola Estés

Index

CPD with Radcliffe

You can now use a selection of our books to achieve CPD (Continuing Professional Development) points through directed reading.

We provide a free online form and downloadable certificate for your appraisal portfolio. Look for the CPD logo and register with us at: www.radcliffehealth.com/cpd

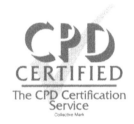